This diary belongs to:

Name: _____

Telephone: _____

Address: _____

GW00503014

_____

In case of emergency please contact:

Name: _____

Telephone: _____

How to use this diary

Record all the information that is relevant to your pain in this diary on daily basis. You may not need to fill out all columns each time. (see example)

Use the image of the human body to mark the exact place of the pain and the type of pain you're having. In the box below the image that you can write down the time period of the pain and description.

Use the rating scale to rate your pain level. A zero (0) means no pain and a ten (10) means worst possible pain. Select the number that best describes your pain.

Take this diary with you to your next appointment. With the help of your diary you can work with your physician to find treatments that work best for you.

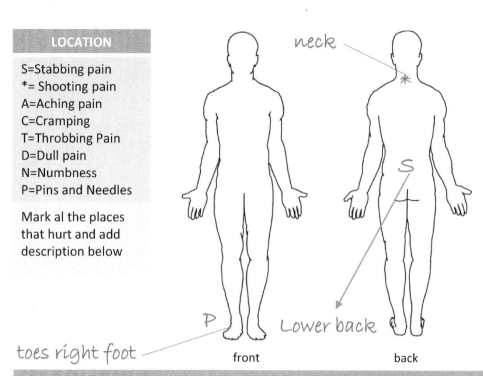

neck

*

S

P

toes right foot

Lower back

front   back

TIME/ DURATION

	Begin	End	Duration		Description
1	8 am	3 pm	5 hrs	6	Shooting pain in neck; left side
2	9 pm	8 am	11 hrs	8	Numb foot during sleep
3	8 pm	??			Pins and needles in toes
4		All Day			Stabbing pain lower back
5					
6					
7					

NOTES (e.g. daily activities, diet, exercise etc.)

Stress at work!

Forgot to take my medicine last night

Mild headache probably because of the humidity,
<u>same as last week</u>!

Example

SYMPTOMS

How well did I sleep?
1 2 3 4 5 6 ⑦ 8 9 10
No rest-------------------------- rested

How energetic do I feel?
1 2 3 4 5 6 ⑦ 8 9 10
Not --------------------------- Very

How anxious do I feel?
1 ② 3 4 5 6 7 8 9 10
Not -------------------------- Extreme

How is my thinking ability
1 2 3 4 5 ⑥ 7 8 9 10
Foggy ------------------------- Clear

How are my bowels?
1 2 3 4 5 6 7 ⑧ 9 10
Constipated------------------------- Loose

How is my appetite affected?
1 ② 3 4 5 6 7 8 9 10
Not------------------------- Very

How is my stress level?
1 2 ③ 4 5 6 7 8 9 10
None------------------------- Extreme

How happy am I ?
1 2 3 4 5 6 7 ⑧ 9 10
Not------------------------- Very

Overall pain level?
1 2 3 ④ 5 6 7 8 9 10
Low------------------------- High

Feeling worried
1 2 3 4 ⑤ 6 7 8 9 10

TRIGGERS

☐ posture	☐ insomnia	☒ humidity	☒ stairs
☐ sleeping	☐ stress	☐ air pressure	☐
☐ exercise	☒ cold/warmth	☐ travel	☐
☒ walking	☐ food	☐ light/sound	☐
☐ weather	☐ lifting	☐ anxiety	☐
☐ allergies	☐ stretching	☐ pms	☐

RELIEF MEASURES

medication	Took a painkiller before sleeping
sleep/rest	
exercise	Yoga exercise helped me relax my muscles
Other	I've stopped drinking coffee... no more headaches now!

LOCATION

S=Stabbing pain
*= Shooting pain
A=Aching pain
C=Cramping
T=Throbbing Pain
D=Dull pain
N=Numbness
P=Pins and Needles

Mark al the places
that hurt and add
description below

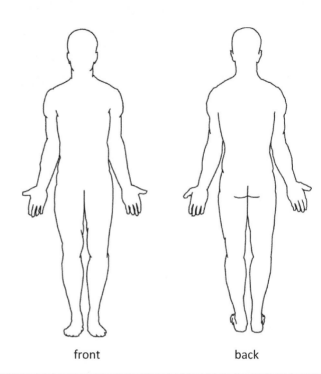

front   back

TIME/ DURATION

	Begin	End	Duration	Description
1				
2				
3				
4				
5				
6				
7				

NOTES (e.g. daily activities, diet, exercise etc.)

SYMPTOMS

How well did I sleep?
1 2 3 4 5 6 7 8 9 10
No rest---------------------------- rested

How energetic do I feel?
1 2 3 4 5 6 7 8 9 10
Not ---------------------------- Very

How anxious do I feel?
1 2 3 4 5 6 7 8 9 10
Not -------------------------- Extreme

How is my thinking ability
1 2 3 4 5 6 7 8 9 10
Foggy -------------------------- Clear

How are my bowels?
1 2 3 4 5 6 7 8 9 10
Constipated------------------------- Loose

How is my appetite affected?
1 2 3 4 5 6 7 8 9 10
Not---------------------------- Very

How is my stress level?
1 2 3 4 5 6 7 8 9 10
None------------------------- Extreme

How happy am I ?
1 2 3 4 5 6 7 8 9 10
Not---------------------------- Very

Overall pain level?
1 2 3 4 5 6 7 8 9 10
Low--------------------------- High

....
1 2 3 4 5 6 7 8 9 10

TRIGGERS

☐ posture	☐ insomnia	☐ humidity	☐
☐ sleeping	☐ stress	☐ air pressure	☐
☐ exercise	☐ cold/warmth	☐ travel	☐
☐ walking	☐ food	☐ light/sound	☐
☐ weather	☐ lifting	☐ anxiety	☐
☐ allergies	☐ stretching	☐ pms	☐

RELIEF MEASURES

medication

sleep/rest

exercise

Other

LOCATION

S=Stabbing pain
*= Shooting pain
A=Aching pain
C=Cramping
T=Throbbing Pain
D=Dull pain
N=Numbness
P=Pins and Needles

Mark al the places
that hurt and add
description below

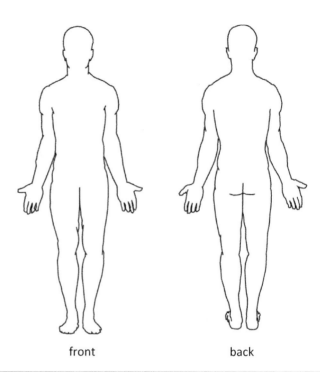

front   back

TIME/ DURATION

	Begin	End	Duration	Description
1				
2				
3				
4				
5				
6				
7				

NOTES (e.g. daily activities, diet, exercise etc.)

SYMPTOMS

How well did I sleep?
1 2 3 4 5 6 7 8 9 10
No rest--------------------------- rested

How energetic do I feel?
1 2 3 4 5 6 7 8 9 10
Not --------------------------- Very

How anxious do I feel?
1 2 3 4 5 6 7 8 9 10
Not --------------------------- Extreme

How is my thinking ability
1 2 3 4 5 6 7 8 9 10
Foggy --------------------------- Clear

How are my bowels?
1 2 3 4 5 6 7 8 9 10
Constipated------------------------- Loose

How is my appetite affected?
1 2 3 4 5 6 7 8 9 10
Not--------------------------- Very

How is my stress level?
1 2 3 4 5 6 7 8 9 10
None------------------------- Extreme

How happy am I ?
1 2 3 4 5 6 7 8 9 10
Not--------------------------- Very

Overall pain level?
1 2 3 4 5 6 7 8 9 10
Low------------------------- High

....
1 2 3 4 5 6 7 8 9 10

TRIGGERS

☐ posture	☐ insomnia	☐ humidity	☐
☐ sleeping	☐ stress	☐ air pressure	☐
☐ exercise	☐ cold/warmth	☐ travel	☐
☐ walking	☐ food	☐ light/sound	☐
☐ weather	☐ lifting	☐ anxiety	☐
☐ allergies	☐ stretching	☐ pms	☐

RELIEF MEASURES

medication

sleep/rest

exercise

Other

LOCATION

S=Stabbing pain
*= Shooting pain
A=Aching pain
C=Cramping
T=Throbbing Pain
D=Dull pain
N=Numbness
P=Pins and Needles

Mark al the places
that hurt and add
description below

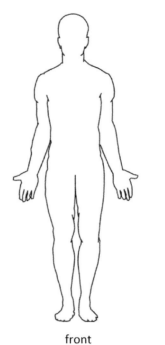

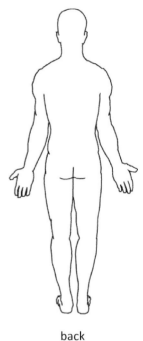

front   back

TIME/ DURATION

	Begin	End	Duration	Description
1				
2				
3				
4				
5				
6				
7				

NOTES (e.g. daily activities, diet, exercise etc.)

DATE	

SYMPTOMS

How well did I sleep?	How energetic do I feel?
1 2 3 4 5 6 7 8 9 10	1 2 3 4 5 6 7 8 9 10
No rest---------------------------- rested	Not --------------------------- Very

How anxious do I feel?	How is my thinking ability
1 2 3 4 5 6 7 8 9 10	1 2 3 4 5 6 7 8 9 10
Not -------------------------- Extreme	Foggy -------------------------- Clear

How are my bowels?	How is my appetite affected?
1 2 3 4 5 6 7 8 9 10	1 2 3 4 5 6 7 8 9 10
Constipated------------------------- Loose	Not--------------------------- Very

How is my stress level?	How happy am I ?
1 2 3 4 5 6 7 8 9 10	1 2 3 4 5 6 7 8 9 10
None------------------------- Extreme	Not--------------------------- Very

Overall pain level?	....
1 2 3 4 5 6 7 8 9 10	1 2 3 4 5 6 7 8 9 10
Low-------------------------- High	--------------------------

TRIGGERS

☐ posture	☐ insomnia	☐ humidity	☐
☐ sleeping	☐ stress	☐ air pressure	☐
☐ exercise	☐ cold/warmth	☐ travel	☐
☐ walking	☐ food	☐ light/sound	☐
☐ weather	☐ lifting	☐ anxiety	☐
☐ allergies	☐ stretching	☐ pms	☐

RELIEF MEASURES

medication	
sleep/rest	
exercise	
Other	

LOCATION

S=Stabbing pain
*= Shooting pain
A=Aching pain
C=Cramping
T=Throbbing Pain
D=Dull pain
N=Numbness
P=Pins and Needles

Mark al the places
that hurt and add
description below

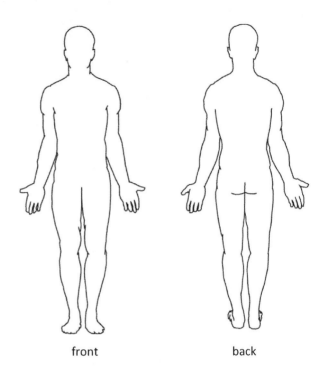

front   back

TIME/ DURATION

	Begin	End	Duration	Description
1				
2				
3				
4				
5				
6				
7				

NOTES (e.g. daily activities, diet, exercise etc.)

SYMPTOMS

How well did I sleep?
1 2 3 4 5 6 7 8 9 10
No rest---------------------------- rested

How energetic do I feel?
1 2 3 4 5 6 7 8 9 10
Not ---------------------------- Very

How anxious do I feel?
1 2 3 4 5 6 7 8 9 10
Not -------------------------- Extreme

How is my thinking ability
1 2 3 4 5 6 7 8 9 10
Foggy -------------------------- Clear

How are my bowels?
1 2 3 4 5 6 7 8 9 10
Constipated------------------------- Loose

How is my appetite affected?
1 2 3 4 5 6 7 8 9 10
Not---------------------------- Very

How is my stress level?
1 2 3 4 5 6 7 8 9 10
None------------------------- Extreme

How happy am I ?
1 2 3 4 5 6 7 8 9 10
Not-------------------------- Very

Overall pain level?
1 2 3 4 5 6 7 8 9 10
Low-------------------------- High

....
1 2 3 4 5 6 7 8 9 10

TRIGGERS

- ☐ posture
- ☐ sleeping
- ☐ exercise
- ☐ walking
- ☐ weather
- ☐ allergies

- ☐ insomnia
- ☐ stress
- ☐ cold/warmth
- ☐ food
- ☐ lifting
- ☐ stretching

- ☐ humidity
- ☐ air pressure
- ☐ travel
- ☐ light/sound
- ☐ anxiety
- ☐ pms

- ☐
- ☐
- ☐
- ☐
- ☐
- ☐

RELIEF MEASURES

medication

sleep/rest

exercise

Other

LOCATION

S=Stabbing pain
*= Shooting pain
A=Aching pain
C=Cramping
T=Throbbing Pain
D=Dull pain
N=Numbness
P=Pins and Needles

Mark al the places
that hurt and add
description below

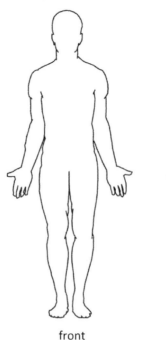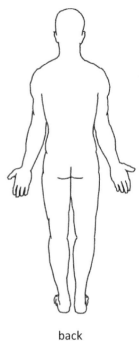

front   back

TIME/ DURATION

	Begin	End	Duration	Description
1				
2				
3				
4				
5				
6				
7				

NOTES (e.g. daily activities, diet, exercise etc.)

SYMPTOMS

How well did I sleep?	How energetic do I feel?
1 2 3 4 5 6 7 8 9 10	1 2 3 4 5 6 7 8 9 10
No rest------------------------- rested	Not -------------------------- Very

How anxious do I feel?	How is my thinking ability
1 2 3 4 5 6 7 8 9 10	1 2 3 4 5 6 7 8 9 10
Not -------------------------- Extreme	Foggy -------------------------- Clear

How are my bowels?	How is my appetite affected?
1 2 3 4 5 6 7 8 9 10	1 2 3 4 5 6 7 8 9 10
Constipated------------------------- Loose	Not-------------------------- Very

How is my stress level?	How happy am I ?
1 2 3 4 5 6 7 8 9 10	1 2 3 4 5 6 7 8 9 10
None------------------------ Extreme	Not-------------------------- Very

Overall pain level?	....
1 2 3 4 5 6 7 8 9 10	1 2 3 4 5 6 7 8 9 10
Low-------------------------- High	--------------------------

TRIGGERS

☐ posture	☐ insomnia	☐ humidity	☐
☐ sleeping	☐ stress	☐ air pressure	☐
☐ exercise	☐ cold/warmth	☐ travel	☐
☐ walking	☐ food	☐ light/sound	☐
☐ weather	☐ lifting	☐ anxiety	☐
☐ allergies	☐ stretching	☐ pms	☐

RELIEF MEASURES

medication	
sleep/rest	
exercise	
Other	

S=Stabbing pain
*= Shooting pain
A=Aching pain
C=Cramping
T=Throbbing Pain
D=Dull pain
N=Numbness
P=Pins and Needles

Mark al the places
that hurt and add
description below

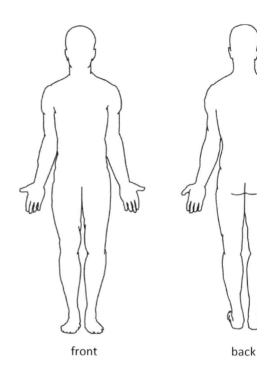

front   back

TIME/ DURATION

	Begin	End	Duration	Description
1				
2				
3				
4				
5				
6				
7				

NOTES (e.g. daily activities, diet, exercise etc.)

DATE	

SYMPTOMS

How well did I sleep?

1 2 3 4 5 6 7 8 9 10

No rest-------------------------- rested

How energetic do I feel?

1 2 3 4 5 6 7 8 9 10

Not -------------------------- Very

How anxious do I feel?

1 2 3 4 5 6 7 8 9 10

Not -------------------------- Extreme

How is my thinking ability

1 2 3 4 5 6 7 8 9 10

Foggy -------------------------- Clear

How are my bowels?

1 2 3 4 5 6 7 8 9 10

Constipated------------------------ Loose

How is my appetite affected?

1 2 3 4 5 6 7 8 9 10

Not-------------------------- Very

How is my stress level?

1 2 3 4 5 6 7 8 9 10

None------------------------ Extreme

How happy am I ?

1 2 3 4 5 6 7 8 9 10

Not-------------------------- Very

Overall pain level?

1 2 3 4 5 6 7 8 9 10

Low------------------------ High

....

1 2 3 4 5 6 7 8 9 10

TRIGGERS

☐ posture   ☐ insomnia   ☐ humidity   ☐

☐ sleeping   ☐ stress   ☐ air pressure ☐

☐ exercise   ☐ cold/warmth   ☐ travel   ☐

☐ walking   ☐ food   ☐ light/sound   ☐

☐ weather   ☐ lifting   ☐ anxiety   ☐

☐ allergies   ☐ stretching   ☐ pms   ☐

RELIEF MEASURES

medication

sleep/rest

exercise

Other

S=Stabbing pain
*= Shooting pain
A=Aching pain
C=Cramping
T=Throbbing Pain
D=Dull pain
N=Numbness
P=Pins and Needles

Mark al the places
that hurt and add
description below

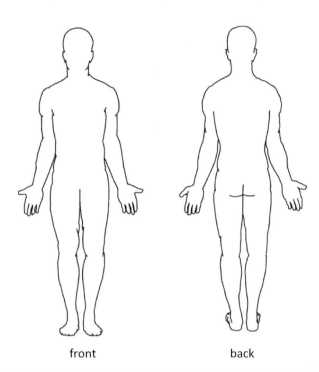

front   back

TIME/ DURATION

	Begin	End	Duration	Description
1				
2				
3				
4				
5				
6				
7				

NOTES (e.g. daily activities, diet, exercise etc.)

SYMPTOMS

How well did I sleep?	How energetic do I feel?
1 2 3 4 5 6 7 8 9 10	1 2 3 4 5 6 7 8 9 10
No rest--------------------------- rested	Not --------------------------- Very

How anxious do I feel?	How is my thinking ability
1 2 3 4 5 6 7 8 9 10	1 2 3 4 5 6 7 8 9 10
Not --------------------------- Extreme	Foggy --------------------------- Clear

How are my bowels?	How is my appetite affected?
1 2 3 4 5 6 7 8 9 10	1 2 3 4 5 6 7 8 9 10
Constipated-------------------------- Loose	Not--------------------------- Very

How is my stress level?	How happy am I ?
1 2 3 4 5 6 7 8 9 10	1 2 3 4 5 6 7 8 9 10
None------------------------- Extreme	Not--------------------------- Very

Overall pain level?	....
1 2 3 4 5 6 7 8 9 10	1 2 3 4 5 6 7 8 9 10
Low-------------------------- High	---------------------------

TRIGGERS

☐ posture	☐ insomnia	☐ humidity	☐
☐ sleeping	☐ stress	☐ air pressure	☐
☐ exercise	☐ cold/warmth	☐ travel	☐
☐ walking	☐ food	☐ light/sound	☐
☐ weather	☐ lifting	☐ anxiety	☐
☐ allergies	☐ stretching	☐ pms	☐

RELIEF MEASURES

medication	
sleep/rest	
exercise	
Other	

S=Stabbing pain
*= Shooting pain
A=Aching pain
C=Cramping
T=Throbbing Pain
D=Dull pain
N=Numbness
P=Pins and Needles

Mark al the places
that hurt and add
description below

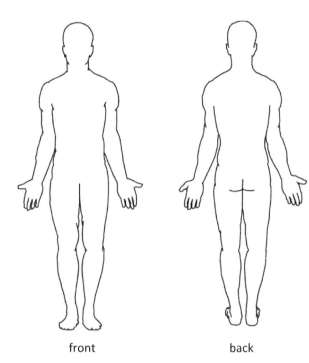

front   back

TIME/ DURATION

	Begin	End	Duration	Description
1				
2				
3				
4				
5				
6				
7				

NOTES (e.g. daily activities, diet, exercise etc.)

DATE	

SYMPTOMS

How well did I sleep?
1 2 3 4 5 6 7 8 9 10
No rest--------------------------- rested

How energetic do I feel?
1 2 3 4 5 6 7 8 9 10
Not --------------------------- Very

How anxious do I feel?
1 2 3 4 5 6 7 8 9 10
Not -------------------------- Extreme

How is my thinking ability
1 2 3 4 5 6 7 8 9 10
Foggy -------------------------- Clear

How are my bowels?
1 2 3 4 5 6 7 8 9 10
Constipated------------------------- Loose

How is my appetite affected?
1 2 3 4 5 6 7 8 9 10
Not--------------------------- Very

How is my stress level?
1 2 3 4 5 6 7 8 9 10
None------------------------- Extreme

How happy am I ?
1 2 3 4 5 6 7 8 9 10
Not--------------------------- Very

Overall pain level?
1 2 3 4 5 6 7 8 9 10
Low------------------------- High

....
1 2 3 4 5 6 7 8 9 10

TRIGGERS

☐ posture	☐ insomnia	☐ humidity	☐
☐ sleeping	☐ stress	☐ air pressure	☐
☐ exercise	☐ cold/warmth	☐ travel	☐
☐ walking	☐ food	☐ light/sound	☐
☐ weather	☐ lifting	☐ anxiety	☐
☐ allergies	☐ stretching	☐ pms	☐

RELIEF MEASURES

medication	
sleep/rest	
exercise	
Other	

LOCATION

S=Stabbing pain
*= Shooting pain
A=Aching pain
C=Cramping
T=Throbbing Pain
D=Dull pain
N=Numbness
P=Pins and Needles

Mark al the places
that hurt and add
description below

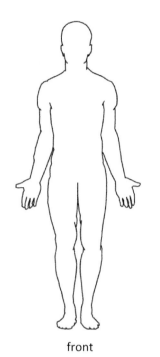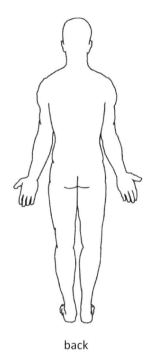

front   back

TIME/ DURATION

	Begin	End	Duration	Description
1				
2				
3				
4				
5				
6				
7				

NOTES (e.g. daily activities, diet, exercise etc.)

SYMPTOMS

How well did I sleep?
1 2 3 4 5 6 7 8 9 10
No rest--------------------------- rested

How energetic do I feel?
1 2 3 4 5 6 7 8 9 10
Not --------------------------- Very

How anxious do I feel?
1 2 3 4 5 6 7 8 9 10
Not -------------------------- Extreme

How is my thinking ability
1 2 3 4 5 6 7 8 9 10
Foggy ------------------------- Clear

How are my bowels?
1 2 3 4 5 6 7 8 9 10
Constipated------------------------- Loose

How is my appetite affected?
1 2 3 4 5 6 7 8 9 10
Not--------------------------- Very

How is my stress level?
1 2 3 4 5 6 7 8 9 10
None------------------------- Extreme

How happy am I ?
1 2 3 4 5 6 7 8 9 10
Not--------------------------- Very

Overall pain level?
1 2 3 4 5 6 7 8 9 10
Low------------------------- High

....
1 2 3 4 5 6 7 8 9 10

TRIGGERS

☐ posture	☐ insomnia	☐ humidity	☐
☐ sleeping	☐ stress	☐ air pressure	☐
☐ exercise	☐ cold/warmth	☐ travel	☐
☐ walking	☐ food	☐ light/sound	☐
☐ weather	☐ lifting	☐ anxiety	☐
☐ allergies	☐ stretching	☐ pms	☐

RELIEF MEASURES

medication	
sleep/rest	
exercise	
Other	

LOCATION

S=Stabbing pain
*= Shooting pain
A=Aching pain
C=Cramping
T=Throbbing Pain
D=Dull pain
N=Numbness
P=Pins and Needles

Mark al the places
that hurt and add
description below

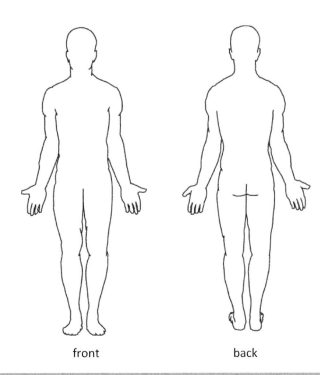

front   back

TIME/ DURATION

	Begin	End	Duration	Description
1				
2				
3				
4				
5				
6				
7				

NOTES (e.g. daily activities, diet, exercise etc.)

SYMPTOMS

How well did I sleep?	How energetic do I feel?
1 2 3 4 5 6 7 8 9 10	1 2 3 4 5 6 7 8 9 10
No rest--------------------------- rested	Not --------------------------- Very

How anxious do I feel?	How is my thinking ability
1 2 3 4 5 6 7 8 9 10	1 2 3 4 5 6 7 8 9 10
Not -------------------------- Extreme	Foggy -------------------------- Clear

How are my bowels?	How is my appetite affected?
1 2 3 4 5 6 7 8 9 10	1 2 3 4 5 6 7 8 9 10
Constipated------------------------ Loose	Not--------------------------- Very

How is my stress level?	How happy am I ?
1 2 3 4 5 6 7 8 9 10	1 2 3 4 5 6 7 8 9 10
None------------------------ Extreme	Not------------------------ Very

Overall pain level?	....
1 2 3 4 5 6 7 8 9 10	1 2 3 4 5 6 7 8 9 10
Low-------------------------- High	--------------------------

TRIGGERS

☐ posture	☐ insomnia	☐ humidity	☐
☐ sleeping	☐ stress	☐ air pressure	☐
☐ exercise	☐ cold/warmth	☐ travel	☐
☐ walking	☐ food	☐ light/sound	☐
☐ weather	☐ lifting	☐ anxiety	☐
☐ allergies	☐ stretching	☐ pms	☐

RELIEF MEASURES

medication

sleep/rest

exercise

Other

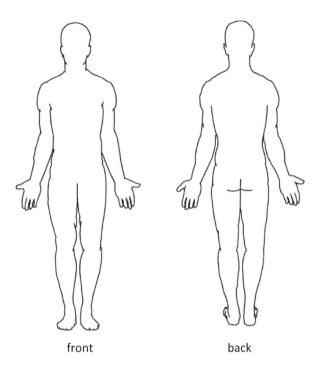

front   back

	Begin	End	Duration	Description
TIME/ DURATION				
1				
2				
3				
4				
5				
6				
7				

NOTES (e.g. daily activities, diet, exercise etc.)

DATE	

SYMPTOMS

How well did I sleep?	How energetic do I feel?
1 2 3 4 5 6 7 8 9 10	1 2 3 4 5 6 7 8 9 10
No rest------------------------- rested	Not -------------------------- Very

How anxious do I feel?	How is my thinking ability
1 2 3 4 5 6 7 8 9 10	1 2 3 4 5 6 7 8 9 10
Not -------------------------- Extreme	Foggy -------------------------- Clear

How are my bowels?	How is my appetite affected?
1 2 3 4 5 6 7 8 9 10	1 2 3 4 5 6 7 8 9 10
Constipated------------------------- Loose	Not-------------------------- Very

How is my stress level?	How happy am I ?
1 2 3 4 5 6 7 8 9 10	1 2 3 4 5 6 7 8 9 10
None------------------------- Extreme	Not------------------------- Very

Overall pain level?	....
1 2 3 4 5 6 7 8 9 10	1 2 3 4 5 6 7 8 9 10
Low------------------------- High	-------------------------

TRIGGERS

☐ posture	☐ insomnia	☐ humidity	☐
☐ sleeping	☐ stress	☐ air pressure	☐
☐ exercise	☐ cold/warmth	☐ travel	☐
☐ walking	☐ food	☐ light/sound	☐
☐ weather	☐ lifting	☐ anxiety	☐
☐ allergies	☐ stretching	☐ pms	☐

RELIEF MEASURES

medication	
sleep/rest	
exercise	
Other	

LOCATION

S=Stabbing pain
*= Shooting pain
A=Aching pain
C=Cramping
T=Throbbing Pain
D=Dull pain
N=Numbness
P=Pins and Needles

Mark al the places
that hurt and add
description below

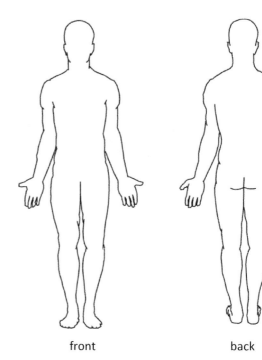

front   back

TIME/ DURATION

	Begin	End	Duration	Description
1				
2				
3				
4				
5				
6				
7				

NOTES (e.g. daily activities, diet, exercise etc.)

DATE	

SYMPTOMS

How well did I sleep?
1 2 3 4 5 6 7 8 9 10
No rest--------------------------- rested

How energetic do I feel?
1 2 3 4 5 6 7 8 9 10
Not --------------------------- Very

How anxious do I feel?
1 2 3 4 5 6 7 8 9 10
Not -------------------------- Extreme

How is my thinking ability
1 2 3 4 5 6 7 8 9 10
Foggy -------------------------- Clear

How are my bowels?
1 2 3 4 5 6 7 8 9 10
Constipated------------------------- Loose

How is my appetite affected?
1 2 3 4 5 6 7 8 9 10
Not------------------------- Very

How is my stress level?
1 2 3 4 5 6 7 8 9 10
None------------------------- Extreme

How happy am I ?
1 2 3 4 5 6 7 8 9 10
Not------------------------- Very

Overall pain level?
1 2 3 4 5 6 7 8 9 10
Low------------------------- High

....
1 2 3 4 5 6 7 8 9 10

TRIGGERS

☐ posture	☐ insomnia	☐ humidity	☐
☐ sleeping	☐ stress	☐ air pressure	☐
☐ exercise	☐ cold/warmth	☐ travel	☐
☐ walking	☐ food	☐ light/sound	☐
☐ weather	☐ lifting	☐ anxiety	☐
☐ allergies	☐ stretching	☐ pms	☐

RELIEF MEASURES

medication	
sleep/rest	
exercise	
Other	

S=Stabbing pain
*= Shooting pain
A=Aching pain
C=Cramping
T=Throbbing Pain
D=Dull pain
N=Numbness
P=Pins and Needles

Mark al the places
that hurt and add
description below

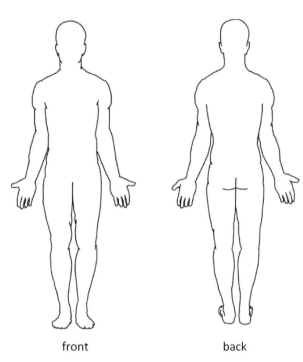

front   back

TIME/ DURATION

	Begin	End	Duration	Description
1				
2				
3				
4				
5				
6				
7				

NOTES (e.g. daily activities, diet, exercise etc.)

DATE	

How well did I sleep?
1 2 3 4 5 6 7 8 9 10
No rest--------------------------- rested

How energetic do I feel?
1 2 3 4 5 6 7 8 9 10
Not --------------------------- Very

How anxious do I feel?
1 2 3 4 5 6 7 8 9 10
Not --------------------------- Extreme

How is my thinking ability
1 2 3 4 5 6 7 8 9 10
Foggy --------------------------- Clear

How are my bowels?
1 2 3 4 5 6 7 8 9 10
Constipated------------------------- Loose

How is my appetite affected?
1 2 3 4 5 6 7 8 9 10
Not--------------------------- Very

How is my stress level?
1 2 3 4 5 6 7 8 9 10
None------------------------- Extreme

How happy am I ?
1 2 3 4 5 6 7 8 9 10
Not--------------------------- Very

Overall pain level?
1 2 3 4 5 6 7 8 9 10
Low------------------------- High

....
1 2 3 4 5 6 7 8 9 10

TRIGGERS

- [ ] posture
- [ ] sleeping
- [ ] exercise
- [ ] walking
- [ ] weather
- [ ] allergies

- [ ] insomnia
- [ ] stress
- [ ] cold/warmth
- [ ] food
- [ ] lifting
- [ ] stretching

- [ ] humidity
- [ ] air pressure
- [ ] travel
- [ ] light/sound
- [ ] anxiety
- [ ] pms

- [ ]
- [ ]
- [ ]
- [ ]
- [ ]
- [ ]

RELIEF MEASURES

medication

sleep/rest

exercise

Other

LOCATION

S=Stabbing pain
*= Shooting pain
A=Aching pain
C=Cramping
T=Throbbing Pain
D=Dull pain
N=Numbness
P=Pins and Needles

Mark al the places
that hurt and add
description below

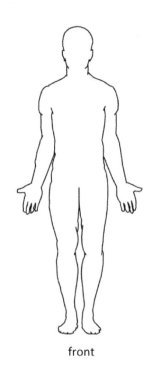 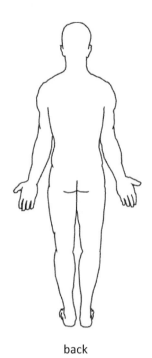

front   back

TIME/ DURATION

	Begin	End	Duration	Description
1				
2				
3				
4				
5				
6				
7				

NOTES (e.g. daily activities, diet, exercise etc.)

SYMPTOMS

How well did I sleep?
1 2 3 4 5 6 7 8 9 10
No rest---------------------------- rested

How energetic do I feel?
1 2 3 4 5 6 7 8 9 10
Not ---------------------------- Very

How anxious do I feel?
1 2 3 4 5 6 7 8 9 10
Not ---------------------------- Extreme

How is my thinking ability
1 2 3 4 5 6 7 8 9 10
Foggy ---------------------------- Clear

How are my bowels?
1 2 3 4 5 6 7 8 9 10
Constipated------------------------- Loose

How is my appetite affected?
1 2 3 4 5 6 7 8 9 10
Not---------------------------- Very

How is my stress level?
1 2 3 4 5 6 7 8 9 10
None------------------------- Extreme

How happy am I ?
1 2 3 4 5 6 7 8 9 10
Not---------------------------- Very

Overall pain level?
1 2 3 4 5 6 7 8 9 10
Low------------------------- High

....
1 2 3 4 5 6 7 8 9 10

TRIGGERS

☐ posture	☐ insomnia	☐ humidity	☐
☐ sleeping	☐ stress	☐ air pressure	☐
☐ exercise	☐ cold/warmth	☐ travel	☐
☐ walking	☐ food	☐ light/sound	☐
☐ weather	☐ lifting	☐ anxiety	☐
☐ allergies	☐ stretching	☐ pms	☐

RELIEF MEASURES

medication

sleep/rest

exercise

Other

S=Stabbing pain
*= Shooting pain
A=Aching pain
C=Cramping
T=Throbbing Pain
D=Dull pain
N=Numbness
P=Pins and Needles

Mark al the places
that hurt and add
description below

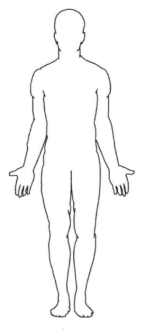 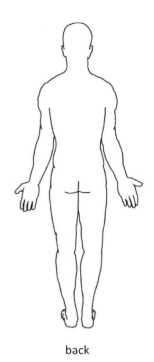

front   back

TIME/ DURATION

	Begin	End	Duration	Description
1				
2				
3				
4				
5				
6				
7				

NOTES (e.g. daily activities, diet, exercise etc.)

SYMPTOMS

How well did I sleep?
1   2   3   4   5   6   7   8   9   10
No rest--------------------------- rested

How energetic do I feel?
1   2   3   4   5   6   7   8   9   10
Not --------------------------- Very

How anxious do I feel?
1   2   3   4   5   6   7   8   9   10
Not --------------------------- Extreme

How is my thinking ability
1   2   3   4   5   6   7   8   9   10
Foggy --------------------------- Clear

How are my bowels?
1   2   3   4   5   6   7   8   9   10
Constipated------------------------ Loose

How is my appetite affected?
1   2   3   4   5   6   7   8   9   10
Not--------------------------- Very

How is my stress level?
1   2   3   4   5   6   7   8   9   10
None------------------------ Extreme

How happy am I ?
1   2   3   4   5   6   7   8   9   10
Not--------------------------- Very

Overall pain level?
1   2   3   4   5   6   7   8   9   10
Low------------------------- High

....
1   2   3   4   5   6   7   8   9   10

TRIGGERS

☐ posture	☐ insomnia	☐ humidity	☐
☐ sleeping	☐ stress	☐ air pressure	☐
☐ exercise	☐ cold/warmth	☐ travel	☐
☐ walking	☐ food	☐ light/sound	☐
☐ weather	☐ lifting	☐ anxiety	☐
☐ allergies	☐ stretching	☐ pms	☐

RELIEF MEASURES

medication

sleep/rest

exercise

Other

LOCATION

S=Stabbing pain
*= Shooting pain
A=Aching pain
C=Cramping
T=Throbbing Pain
D=Dull pain
N=Numbness
P=Pins and Needles

Mark al the places
that hurt and add
description below

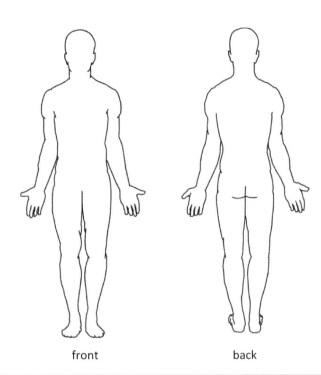

front   back

TIME/ DURATION

	Begin	End	Duration	Description
1				
2				
3				
4				
5				
6				
7				

NOTES (e.g. daily activities, diet, exercise etc.)

SYMPTOMS

How well did I sleep?	How energetic do I feel?
1 2 3 4 5 6 7 8 9 10	1 2 3 4 5 6 7 8 9 10
No rest-------------------------- rested	Not --------------------------- Very

How anxious do I feel?	How is my thinking ability
1 2 3 4 5 6 7 8 9 10	1 2 3 4 5 6 7 8 9 10
Not ----------------------- Extreme	Foggy -------------------------- Clear

How are my bowels?	How is my appetite affected?
1 2 3 4 5 6 7 8 9 10	1 2 3 4 5 6 7 8 9 10
Constipated------------------------- Loose	Not-------------------------- Very

How is my stress level?	How happy am I ?
1 2 3 4 5 6 7 8 9 10	1 2 3 4 5 6 7 8 9 10
None------------------------ Extreme	Not-------------------------- Very

Overall pain level?	....
1 2 3 4 5 6 7 8 9 10	1 2 3 4 5 6 7 8 9 10
Low------------------------- High	--------------------------

TRIGGERS

☐ posture	☐ insomnia	☐ humidity	☐
☐ sleeping	☐ stress	☐ air pressure	☐
☐ exercise	☐ cold/warmth	☐ travel	☐
☐ walking	☐ food	☐ light/sound	☐
☐ weather	☐ lifting	☐ anxiety	☐
☐ allergies	☐ stretching	☐ pms	☐

RELIEF MEASURES

medication

sleep/rest

exercise

Other

S=Stabbing pain
*= Shooting pain
A=Aching pain
C=Cramping
T=Throbbing Pain
D=Dull pain
N=Numbness
P=Pins and Needles

Mark al the places
that hurt and add
description below

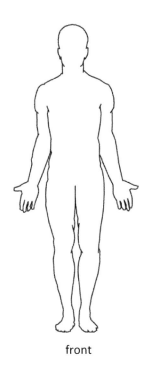 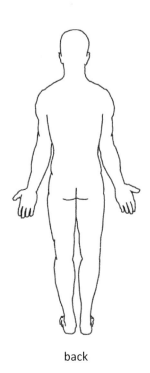

front　　　　　　　　　back

TIME/ DURATION

	Begin	End	Duration	Description
1				
2				
3				
4				
5				
6				
7				

NOTES (e.g. daily activities, diet, exercise etc.)

DATE	

How well did I sleep?

1 2 3 4 5 6 7 8 9 10

No rest-------------------------- rested

How energetic do I feel?

1 2 3 4 5 6 7 8 9 10

Not -------------------------- Very

How anxious do I feel?

1 2 3 4 5 6 7 8 9 10

Not -------------------------- Extreme

How is my thinking ability

1 2 3 4 5 6 7 8 9 10

Foggy -------------------------- Clear

How are my bowels?

1 2 3 4 5 6 7 8 9 10

Constipated------------------------ Loose

How is my appetite affected?

1 2 3 4 5 6 7 8 9 10

Not-------------------------- Very

How is my stress level?

1 2 3 4 5 6 7 8 9 10

None------------------------ Extreme

How happy am I ?

1 2 3 4 5 6 7 8 9 10

Not-------------------------- Very

Overall pain level?

1 2 3 4 5 6 7 8 9 10

Low-------------------------- High

....

1 2 3 4 5 6 7 8 9 10

TRIGGERS

☐ posture	☐ insomnia	☐ humidity	☐
☐ sleeping	☐ stress	☐ air pressure	☐
☐ exercise	☐ cold/warmth	☐ travel	☐
☐ walking	☐ food	☐ light/sound	☐
☐ weather	☐ lifting	☐ anxiety	☐
☐ allergies	☐ stretching	☐ pms	☐

RELIEF MEASURES

medication	
sleep/rest	
exercise	
Other	

S=Stabbing pain
*= Shooting pain
A=Aching pain
C=Cramping
T=Throbbing Pain
D=Dull pain
N=Numbness
P=Pins and Needles

Mark al the places
that hurt and add
description below

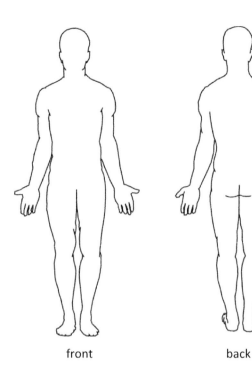

front   back

TIME/ DURATION

	Begin	End	Duration	Description
1				
2				
3				
4				
5				
6				
7				

NOTES (e.g. daily activities, diet, exercise etc.)

SYMPTOMS

How well did I sleep?
1 2 3 4 5 6 7 8 9 10
No rest---------------------------- rested

How energetic do I feel?
1 2 3 4 5 6 7 8 9 10
Not ---------------------------- Very

How anxious do I feel?
1 2 3 4 5 6 7 8 9 10
Not ---------------------------- Extreme

How is my thinking ability
1 2 3 4 5 6 7 8 9 10
Foggy ---------------------------- Clear

How are my bowels?
1 2 3 4 5 6 7 8 9 10
Constipated------------------------- Loose

How is my appetite affected?
1 2 3 4 5 6 7 8 9 10
Not---------------------------- Very

How is my stress level?
1 2 3 4 5 6 7 8 9 10
None------------------------- Extreme

How happy am I ?
1 2 3 4 5 6 7 8 9 10
Not---------------------------- Very

Overall pain level?
1 2 3 4 5 6 7 8 9 10
Low------------------------- High

....
1 2 3 4 5 6 7 8 9 10

TRIGGERS

☐ posture	☐ insomnia	☐ humidity	☐
☐ sleeping	☐ stress	☐ air pressure	☐
☐ exercise	☐ cold/warmth	☐ travel	☐
☐ walking	☐ food	☐ light/sound	☐
☐ weather	☐ lifting	☐ anxiety	☐
☐ allergies	☐ stretching	☐ pms	☐

RELIEF MEASURES

medication

sleep/rest

exercise

Other

LOCATION

S=Stabbing pain
*= Shooting pain
A=Aching pain
C=Cramping
T=Throbbing Pain
D=Dull pain
N=Numbness
P=Pins and Needles

Mark al the places
that hurt and add
description below

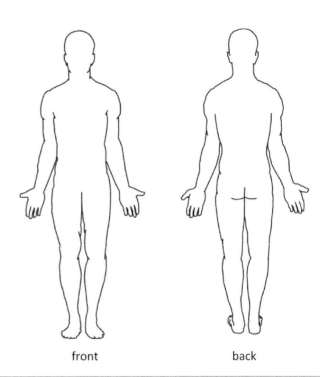

front   back

TIME/ DURATION

	Begin	End	Duration	Description
1				
2				
3				
4				
5				
6				
7				

NOTES (e.g. daily activities, diet, exercise etc.)

SYMPTOMS

How well did I sleep?

1 2 3 4 5 6 7 8 9 10

No rest-------------------------- rested

How energetic do I feel?

1 2 3 4 5 6 7 8 9 10

Not --------------------------- Very

How anxious do I feel?

1 2 3 4 5 6 7 8 9 10

Not -------------------------- Extreme

How is my thinking ability

1 2 3 4 5 6 7 8 9 10

Foggy -------------------------- Clear

How are my bowels?

1 2 3 4 5 6 7 8 9 10

Constipated------------------------ Loose

How is my appetite affected?

1 2 3 4 5 6 7 8 9 10

Not-------------------------- Very

How is my stress level?

1 2 3 4 5 6 7 8 9 10

None------------------------ Extreme

How happy am I ?

1 2 3 4 5 6 7 8 9 10

Not-------------------------- Very

Overall pain level?

1 2 3 4 5 6 7 8 9 10

Low-------------------------- High

....

1 2 3 4 5 6 7 8 9 10

TRIGGERS

- ☐ posture
- ☐ sleeping
- ☐ exercise
- ☐ walking
- ☐ weather
- ☐ allergies

- ☐ insomnia
- ☐ stress
- ☐ cold/warmth
- ☐ food
- ☐ lifting
- ☐ stretching

- ☐ humidity
- ☐ air pressure
- ☐ travel
- ☐ light/sound
- ☐ anxiety
- ☐ pms

- ☐
- ☐
- ☐
- ☐
- ☐
- ☐

RELIEF MEASURES

medication

sleep/rest

exercise

Other

LOCATION

S=Stabbing pain
*= Shooting pain
A=Aching pain
C=Cramping
T=Throbbing Pain
D=Dull pain
N=Numbness
P=Pins and Needles

Mark al the places
that hurt and add
description below

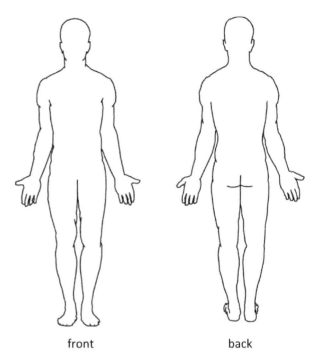

front   back

TIME/ DURATION

	Begin	End	Duration	Description
1				
2				
3				
4				
5				
6				
7				

NOTES (e.g. daily activities, diet, exercise etc.)

DATE	

SYMPTOMS

How well did I sleep?	How energetic do I feel?
1 2 3 4 5 6 7 8 9 10	1 2 3 4 5 6 7 8 9 10
No rest--------------------------- rested	Not --------------------------- Very

How anxious do I feel?	How is my thinking ability
1 2 3 4 5 6 7 8 9 10	1 2 3 4 5 6 7 8 9 10
Not -------------------------- Extreme	Foggy -------------------------- Clear

How are my bowels?	How is my appetite affected?
1 2 3 4 5 6 7 8 9 10	1 2 3 4 5 6 7 8 9 10
Constipated------------------------- Loose	Not--------------------------- Very

How is my stress level?	How happy am I ?
1 2 3 4 5 6 7 8 9 10	1 2 3 4 5 6 7 8 9 10
None------------------------- Extreme	Not--------------------------- Very

Overall pain level?	....
1 2 3 4 5 6 7 8 9 10	1 2 3 4 5 6 7 8 9 10
Low-------------------------- High	--------------------------

TRIGGERS

☐ posture	☐ insomnia	☐ humidity	☐
☐ sleeping	☐ stress	☐ air pressure	☐
☐ exercise	☐ cold/warmth	☐ travel	☐
☐ walking	☐ food	☐ light/sound	☐
☐ weather	☐ lifting	☐ anxiety	☐
☐ allergies	☐ stretching	☐ pms	☐

RELIEF MEASURES

medication	
sleep/rest	
exercise	
Other	

S=Stabbing pain
*= Shooting pain
A=Aching pain
C=Cramping
T=Throbbing Pain
D=Dull pain
N=Numbness
P=Pins and Needles

Mark al the places
that hurt and add
description below

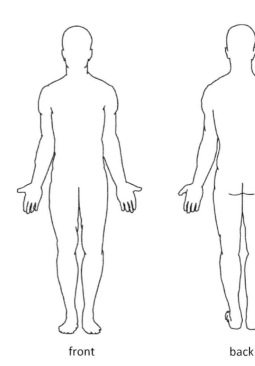

front   back

TIME/ DURATION

	Begin	End	Duration	Description
1				
2				
3				
4				
5				
6				
7				

NOTES (e.g. daily activities, diet, exercise etc.)

DATE	

SYMPTOMS

How well did I sleep?
1 2 3 4 5 6 7 8 9 10
No rest--------------------------- rested

How energetic do I feel?
1 2 3 4 5 6 7 8 9 10
Not --------------------------- Very

How anxious do I feel?
1 2 3 4 5 6 7 8 9 10
Not -------------------------- Extreme

How is my thinking ability
1 2 3 4 5 6 7 8 9 10
Foggy -------------------------- Clear

How are my bowels?
1 2 3 4 5 6 7 8 9 10
Constipated------------------------- Loose

How is my appetite affected?
1 2 3 4 5 6 7 8 9 10
Not--------------------------- Very

How is my stress level?
1 2 3 4 5 6 7 8 9 10
None------------------------- Extreme

How happy am I ?
1 2 3 4 5 6 7 8 9 10
Not--------------------------- Very

Overall pain level?
1 2 3 4 5 6 7 8 9 10
Low-------------------------- High

....
1 2 3 4 5 6 7 8 9 10

TRIGGERS

☐ posture	☐ insomnia	☐ humidity	☐
☐ sleeping	☐ stress	☐ air pressure	☐
☐ exercise	☐ cold/warmth	☐ travel	☐
☐ walking	☐ food	☐ light/sound	☐
☐ weather	☐ lifting	☐ anxiety	☐
☐ allergies	☐ stretching	☐ pms	☐

RELIEF MEASURES

medication	
sleep/rest	
exercise	
Other	

LOCATION

S=Stabbing pain
*= Shooting pain
A=Aching pain
C=Cramping
T=Throbbing Pain
D=Dull pain
N=Numbness
P=Pins and Needles

Mark al the places
that hurt and add
description below

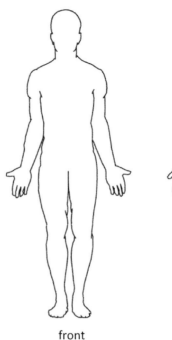

front   back

TIME/ DURATION

	Begin	End	Duration	Description
1				
2				
3				
4				
5				
6				
7				

NOTES (e.g. daily activities, diet, exercise etc.)

DATE	

SYMPTOMS

How well did I sleep?
1 2 3 4 5 6 7 8 9 10
No rest-------------------------- rested

How energetic do I feel?
1 2 3 4 5 6 7 8 9 10
Not --------------------------- Very

How anxious do I feel?
1 2 3 4 5 6 7 8 9 10
Not -------------------------- Extreme

How is my thinking ability
1 2 3 4 5 6 7 8 9 10
Foggy -------------------------- Clear

How are my bowels?
1 2 3 4 5 6 7 8 9 10
Constipated------------------------ Loose

How is my appetite affected?
1 2 3 4 5 6 7 8 9 10
Not-------------------------- Very

How is my stress level?
1 2 3 4 5 6 7 8 9 10
None------------------------ Extreme

How happy am I ?
1 2 3 4 5 6 7 8 9 10
Not-------------------------- Very

Overall pain level?
1 2 3 4 5 6 7 8 9 10
Low-------------------------- High

....
1 2 3 4 5 6 7 8 9 10

TRIGGERS

- [ ] posture
- [ ] sleeping
- [ ] exercise
- [ ] walking
- [ ] weather
- [ ] allergies

- [ ] insomnia
- [ ] stress
- [ ] cold/warmth
- [ ] food
- [ ] lifting
- [ ] stretching

- [ ] humidity
- [ ] air pressure
- [ ] travel
- [ ] light/sound
- [ ] anxiety
- [ ] pms

- [ ]
- [ ]
- [ ]
- [ ]
- [ ]
- [ ]

RELIEF MEASURES

medication

sleep/rest

exercise

Other

LOCATION

S=Stabbing pain
*= Shooting pain
A=Aching pain
C=Cramping
T=Throbbing Pain
D=Dull pain
N=Numbness
P=Pins and Needles

Mark al the places
that hurt and add
description below

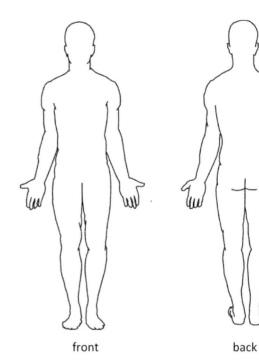

front   back

TIME/ DURATION

	Begin	End	Duration	Description
1				
2				
3				
4				
5				
6				
7				

NOTES (e.g. daily activities, diet, exercise etc.)

SYMPTOMS

How well did I sleep?

1 2 3 4 5 6 7 8 9 10

No rest---------------------------- rested

How energetic do I feel?

1 2 3 4 5 6 7 8 9 10

Not ---------------------------- Very

How anxious do I feel?

1 2 3 4 5 6 7 8 9 10

Not ------------------------- Extreme

How is my thinking ability

1 2 3 4 5 6 7 8 9 10

Foggy -------------------------- Clear

How are my bowels?

1 2 3 4 5 6 7 8 9 10

Constipated------------------------- Loose

How is my appetite affected?

1 2 3 4 5 6 7 8 9 10

Not---------------------------- Very

How is my stress level?

1 2 3 4 5 6 7 8 9 10

None------------------------- Extreme

How happy am I ?

1 2 3 4 5 6 7 8 9 10

Not------------------------- Very

Overall pain level?

1 2 3 4 5 6 7 8 9 10

Low------------------------- High

....

1 2 3 4 5 6 7 8 9 10

TRIGGERS

☐ posture	☐ insomnia	☐ humidity	☐
☐ sleeping	☐ stress	☐ air pressure	☐
☐ exercise	☐ cold/warmth	☐ travel	☐
☐ walking	☐ food	☐ light/sound	☐
☐ weather	☐ lifting	☐ anxiety	☐
☐ allergies	☐ stretching	☐ pms	☐

RELIEF MEASURES

medication

sleep/rest

exercise

Other

S=Stabbing pain
*= Shooting pain
A=Aching pain
C=Cramping
T=Throbbing Pain
D=Dull pain
N=Numbness
P=Pins and Needles

Mark al the places
that hurt and add
description below

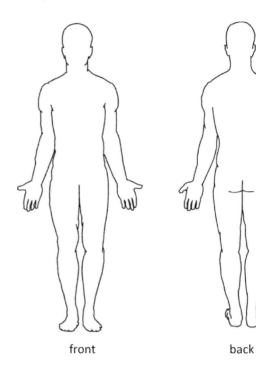

front   back

TIME/ DURATION

	Begin	End	Duration	Description
1				
2				
3				
4				
5				
6				
7				

NOTES (e.g. daily activities, diet, exercise etc.)

SYMPTOMS

How well did I sleep?
1 2 3 4 5 6 7 8 9 10
No rest---------------------------- rested

How energetic do I feel?
1 2 3 4 5 6 7 8 9 10
Not ---------------------------- Very

How anxious do I feel?
1 2 3 4 5 6 7 8 9 10
Not -------------------------- Extreme

How is my thinking ability
1 2 3 4 5 6 7 8 9 10
Foggy -------------------------- Clear

How are my bowels?
1 2 3 4 5 6 7 8 9 10
Constipated------------------------- Loose

How is my appetite affected?
1 2 3 4 5 6 7 8 9 10
Not---------------------------- Very

How is my stress level?
1 2 3 4 5 6 7 8 9 10
None------------------------- Extreme

How happy am I ?
1 2 3 4 5 6 7 8 9 10
Not---------------------------- Very

Overall pain level?
1 2 3 4 5 6 7 8 9 10
Low------------------------- High

....
1 2 3 4 5 6 7 8 9 10

TRIGGERS

☐ posture	☐ insomnia	☐ humidity	☐
☐ sleeping	☐ stress	☐ air pressure	☐
☐ exercise	☐ cold/warmth	☐ travel	☐
☐ walking	☐ food	☐ light/sound	☐
☐ weather	☐ lifting	☐ anxiety	☐
☐ allergies	☐ stretching	☐ pms	☐

RELIEF MEASURES

medication

sleep/rest

exercise

Other

LOCATION

S=Stabbing pain
*= Shooting pain
A=Aching pain
C=Cramping
T=Throbbing Pain
D=Dull pain
N=Numbness
P=Pins and Needles

Mark al the places
that hurt and add
description below

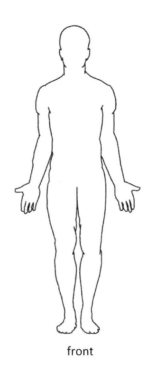
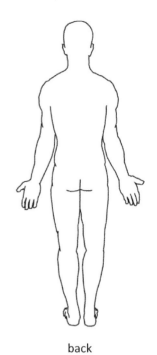

front   back

TIME/ DURATION

	Begin	End	Duration	Description
1				
2				
3				
4				
5				
6				
7				

NOTES (e.g. daily activities, diet, exercise etc.)

SYMPTOMS

How well did I sleep?
1 2 3 4 5 6 7 8 9 10
No rest---------------------------- rested

How energetic do I feel?
1 2 3 4 5 6 7 8 9 10
Not ---------------------------- Very

How anxious do I feel?
1 2 3 4 5 6 7 8 9 10
Not -------------------------- Extreme

How is my thinking ability
1 2 3 4 5 6 7 8 9 10
Foggy ------------------------- Clear

How are my bowels?
1 2 3 4 5 6 7 8 9 10
Constipated------------------------- Loose

How is my appetite affected?
1 2 3 4 5 6 7 8 9 10
Not--------------------------- Very

How is my stress level?
1 2 3 4 5 6 7 8 9 10
None------------------------- Extreme

How happy am I ?
1 2 3 4 5 6 7 8 9 10
Not--------------------------- Very

Overall pain level?
1 2 3 4 5 6 7 8 9 10
Low-------------------------- High

....
1 2 3 4 5 6 7 8 9 10

TRIGGERS

- [ ] posture
- [ ] sleeping
- [ ] exercise
- [ ] walking
- [ ] weather
- [ ] allergies

- [ ] insomnia
- [ ] stress
- [ ] cold/warmth
- [ ] food
- [ ] lifting
- [ ] stretching

- [ ] humidity
- [ ] air pressure
- [ ] travel
- [ ] light/sound
- [ ] anxiety
- [ ] pms

- [ ]
- [ ]
- [ ]
- [ ]
- [ ]
- [ ]

RELIEF MEASURES

medication

sleep/rest

exercise

Other

S=Stabbing pain
*= Shooting pain
A=Aching pain
C=Cramping
T=Throbbing Pain
D=Dull pain
N=Numbness
P=Pins and Needles

Mark al the places
that hurt and add
description below

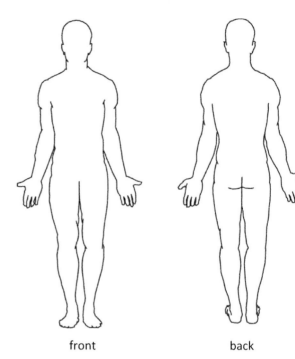

front   back

TIME/ DURATION

	Begin	End	Duration	Description
1				
2				
3				
4				
5				
6				
7				

NOTES (e.g. daily activities, diet, exercise etc.)

SYMPTOMS

How well did I sleep?	How energetic do I feel?
1 2 3 4 5 6 7 8 9 10	1 2 3 4 5 6 7 8 9 10
No rest---------------------------- rested	Not --------------------------- Very

How anxious do I feel?	How is my thinking ability
1 2 3 4 5 6 7 8 9 10	1 2 3 4 5 6 7 8 9 10
Not -------------------------- Extreme	Foggy --------------------------- Clear

How are my bowels?	How is my appetite affected?
1 2 3 4 5 6 7 8 9 10	1 2 3 4 5 6 7 8 9 10
Constipated------------------------ Loose	Not--------------------------- Very

How is my stress level?	How happy am I ?
1 2 3 4 5 6 7 8 9 10	1 2 3 4 5 6 7 8 9 10
None------------------------ Extreme	Not-------------------------- Very

Overall pain level?	....
1 2 3 4 5 6 7 8 9 10	1 2 3 4 5 6 7 8 9 10
Low------------------------- High	---------------------------

TRIGGERS

☐ posture	☐ insomnia	☐ humidity	☐
☐ sleeping	☐ stress	☐ air pressure	☐
☐ exercise	☐ cold/warmth	☐ travel	☐
☐ walking	☐ food	☐ light/sound	☐
☐ weather	☐ lifting	☐ anxiety	☐
☐ allergies	☐ stretching	☐ pms	☐

RELIEF MEASURES

medication	
sleep/rest	
exercise	
Other	

LOCATION

S=Stabbing pain
*= Shooting pain
A=Aching pain
C=Cramping
T=Throbbing Pain
D=Dull pain
N=Numbness
P=Pins and Needles

Mark al the places
that hurt and add
description below

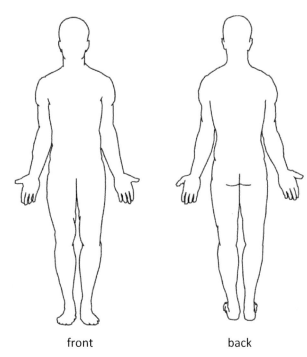

front   back

TIME/ DURATION

	Begin	End	Duration	Description
1				
2				
3				
4				
5				
6				
7				

NOTES (e.g. daily activities, diet, exercise etc.)

DATE	

SYMPTOMS

How well did I sleep?
1 2 3 4 5 6 7 8 9 10
No rest-------------------------- rested

How energetic do I feel?
1 2 3 4 5 6 7 8 9 10
Not -------------------------- Very

How anxious do I feel?
1 2 3 4 5 6 7 8 9 10
Not ------------------------- Extreme

How is my thinking ability
1 2 3 4 5 6 7 8 9 10
Foggy ------------------------- Clear

How are my bowels?
1 2 3 4 5 6 7 8 9 10
Constipated------------------------- Loose

How is my appetite affected?
1 2 3 4 5 6 7 8 9 10
Not------------------------- Very

How is my stress level?
1 2 3 4 5 6 7 8 9 10
None------------------------- Extreme

How happy am I ?
1 2 3 4 5 6 7 8 9 10
Not------------------------- Very

Overall pain level?
1 2 3 4 5 6 7 8 9 10
Low------------------------- High

....
1 2 3 4 5 6 7 8 9 10

TRIGGERS

☐ posture	☐ insomnia	☐ humidity	☐
☐ sleeping	☐ stress	☐ air pressure	☐
☐ exercise	☐ cold/warmth	☐ travel	☐
☐ walking	☐ food	☐ light/sound	☐
☐ weather	☐ lifting	☐ anxiety	☐
☐ allergies	☐ stretching	☐ pms	☐

RELIEF MEASURES

medication	
sleep/rest	
exercise	
Other	

LOCATION

S=Stabbing pain
*= Shooting pain
A=Aching pain
C=Cramping
T=Throbbing Pain
D=Dull pain
N=Numbness
P=Pins and Needles

Mark al the places
that hurt and add
description below

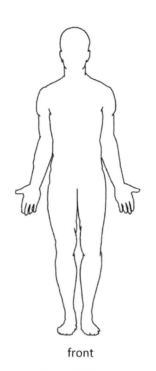
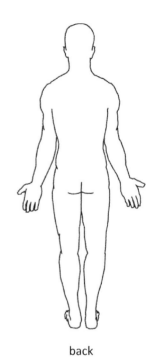

front   back

TIME/ DURATION

	Begin	End	Duration	Description
1				
2				
3				
4				
5				
6				
7				

NOTES (e.g. daily activities, diet, exercise etc.)

DATE	

How well did I sleep?

1 2 3 4 5 6 7 8 9 10

No rest---------------------------- rested

How energetic do I feel?

1 2 3 4 5 6 7 8 9 10

Not ---------------------------- Very

How anxious do I feel?

1 2 3 4 5 6 7 8 9 10

Not ---------------------------- Extreme

How is my thinking ability

1 2 3 4 5 6 7 8 9 10

Foggy ---------------------------- Clear

How are my bowels?

1 2 3 4 5 6 7 8 9 10

Constipated---------------------- Loose

How is my appetite affected?

1 2 3 4 5 6 7 8 9 10

Not---------------------------- Very

How is my stress level?

1 2 3 4 5 6 7 8 9 10

None---------------------- Extreme

How happy am I ?

1 2 3 4 5 6 7 8 9 10

Not---------------------------- Very

Overall pain level?

1 2 3 4 5 6 7 8 9 10

Low---------------------------- High

....

1 2 3 4 5 6 7 8 9 10

TRIGGERS

- ☐ posture
- ☐ sleeping
- ☐ exercise
- ☐ walking
- ☐ weather
- ☐ allergies

- ☐ insomnia
- ☐ stress
- ☐ cold/warmth
- ☐ food
- ☐ lifting
- ☐ stretching

- ☐ humidity
- ☐ air pressure
- ☐ travel
- ☐ light/sound
- ☐ anxiety
- ☐ pms

- ☐
- ☐
- ☐
- ☐
- ☐
- ☐

RELIEF MEASURES

medication

sleep/rest

exercise

Other

LOCATION

S=Stabbing pain
*= Shooting pain
A=Aching pain
C=Cramping
T=Throbbing Pain
D=Dull pain
N=Numbness
P=Pins and Needles

Mark al the places
that hurt and add
description below

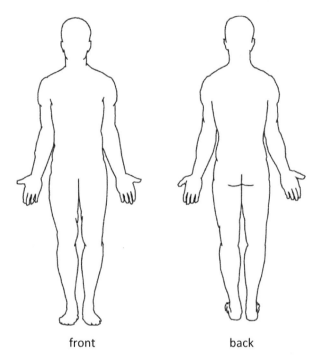

front   back

TIME/ DURATION

	Begin	End	Duration	Description
1				
2				
3				
4				
5				
6				
7				

NOTES (e.g. daily activities, diet, exercise etc.)

SYMPTOMS

How well did I sleep?	How energetic do I feel?
1 2 3 4 5 6 7 8 9 10	1 2 3 4 5 6 7 8 9 10
No rest------------------------- rested	Not -------------------------- Very

How anxious do I feel?	How is my thinking ability
1 2 3 4 5 6 7 8 9 10	1 2 3 4 5 6 7 8 9 10
Not ------------------------ Extreme	Foggy --------------------------- Clear

How are my bowels?	How is my appetite affected?
1 2 3 4 5 6 7 8 9 10	1 2 3 4 5 6 7 8 9 10
Constipated------------------------ Loose	Not-------------------------- Very

How is my stress level?	How happy am I ?
1 2 3 4 5 6 7 8 9 10	1 2 3 4 5 6 7 8 9 10
None------------------------ Extreme	Not-------------------------- Very

Overall pain level?	....
1 2 3 4 5 6 7 8 9 10	1 2 3 4 5 6 7 8 9 10
Low-------------------------- High	--------------------------

TRIGGERS

☐ posture	☐ insomnia	☐ humidity	☐
☐ sleeping	☐ stress	☐ air pressure	☐
☐ exercise	☐ cold/warmth	☐ travel	☐
☐ walking	☐ food	☐ light/sound	☐
☐ weather	☐ lifting	☐ anxiety	☐
☐ allergies	☐ stretching	☐ pms	☐

RELIEF MEASURES

medication	
sleep/rest	
exercise	
Other	

LOCATION

S=Stabbing pain
*= Shooting pain
A=Aching pain
C=Cramping
T=Throbbing Pain
D=Dull pain
N=Numbness
P=Pins and Needles

Mark al the places
that hurt and add
description below

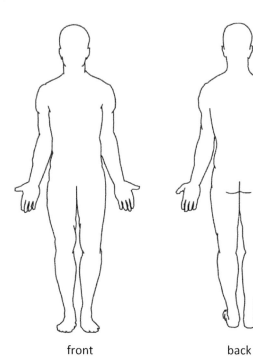

front   back

TIME/ DURATION

	Begin	End	Duration	Description
1				
2				
3				
4				
5				
6				
7				

NOTES (e.g. daily activities, diet, exercise etc.)

SYMPTOMS

How well did I sleep?
1 2 3 4 5 6 7 8 9 10
No rest---------------------------- rested

How energetic do I feel?
1 2 3 4 5 6 7 8 9 10
Not ---------------------------- Very

How anxious do I feel?
1 2 3 4 5 6 7 8 9 10
Not ------------------------- Extreme

How is my thinking ability
1 2 3 4 5 6 7 8 9 10
Foggy ------------------------- Clear

How are my bowels?
1 2 3 4 5 6 7 8 9 10
Constipated------------------------ Loose

How is my appetite affected?
1 2 3 4 5 6 7 8 9 10
Not-------------------------- Very

How is my stress level?
1 2 3 4 5 6 7 8 9 10
None------------------------ Extreme

How happy am I ?
1 2 3 4 5 6 7 8 9 10
Not-------------------------- Very

Overall pain level?
1 2 3 4 5 6 7 8 9 10
Low------------------------- High

....
1 2 3 4 5 6 7 8 9 10

TRIGGERS

☐ posture   ☐ insomnia   ☐ humidity   ☐
☐ sleeping   ☐ stress   ☐ air pressure   ☐
☐ exercise   ☐ cold/warmth   ☐ travel   ☐
☐ walking   ☐ food   ☐ light/sound   ☐
☐ weather   ☐ lifting   ☐ anxiety   ☐
☐ allergies   ☐ stretching   ☐ pms   ☐

RELIEF MEASURES

medication

sleep/rest

exercise

Other

LOCATION

S=Stabbing pain
*= Shooting pain
A=Aching pain
C=Cramping
T=Throbbing Pain
D=Dull pain
N=Numbness
P=Pins and Needles

Mark al the places
that hurt and add
description below

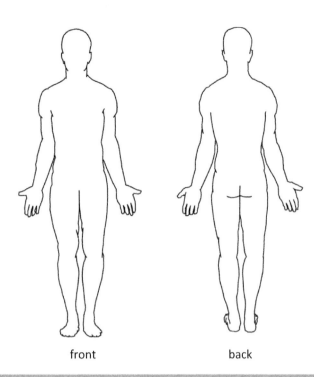

front   back

TIME/ DURATION

	Begin	End	Duration	Description
1				
2				
3				
4				
5				
6				
7				

NOTES (e.g. daily activities, diet, exercise etc.)

SYMPTOMS

How well did I sleep?

1 2 3 4 5 6 7 8 9 10

No rest--------------------------- rested

How energetic do I feel?

1 2 3 4 5 6 7 8 9 10

Not --------------------------- Very

How anxious do I feel?

1 2 3 4 5 6 7 8 9 10

Not -------------------------- Extreme

How is my thinking ability

1 2 3 4 5 6 7 8 9 10

Foggy -------------------------- Clear

How are my bowels?

1 2 3 4 5 6 7 8 9 10

Constipated------------------------ Loose

How is my appetite affected?

1 2 3 4 5 6 7 8 9 10

Not--------------------------- Very

How is my stress level?

1 2 3 4 5 6 7 8 9 10

None------------------------- Extreme

How happy am I ?

1 2 3 4 5 6 7 8 9 10

Not--------------------------- Very

Overall pain level?

1 2 3 4 5 6 7 8 9 10

Low-------------------------- High

....

1 2 3 4 5 6 7 8 9 10

TRIGGERS

☐ posture   ☐ insomnia   ☐ humidity   ☐

☐ sleeping   ☐ stress   ☐ air pressure   ☐

☐ exercise   ☐ cold/warmth   ☐ travel   ☐

☐ walking   ☐ food   ☐ light/sound   ☐

☐ weather   ☐ lifting   ☐ anxiety   ☐

☐ allergies   ☐ stretching   ☐ pms   ☐

RELIEF MEASURES

medication

sleep/rest

exercise

Other

LOCATION

S=Stabbing pain
*= Shooting pain
A=Aching pain
C=Cramping
T=Throbbing Pain
D=Dull pain
N=Numbness
P=Pins and Needles

Mark al the places
that hurt and add
description below

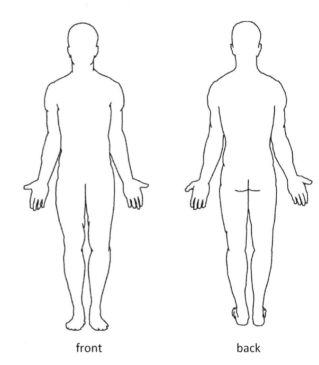

front   back

TIME/ DURATION

	Begin	End	Duration	Description
1				
2				
3				
4				
5				
6				
7				

NOTES (e.g. daily activities, diet, exercise etc.)

SYMPTOMS

How well did I sleep?	How energetic do I feel?
1 2 3 4 5 6 7 8 9 10	1 2 3 4 5 6 7 8 9 10
No rest-------------------------- rested	Not -------------------------- Very

How anxious do I feel?	How is my thinking ability
1 2 3 4 5 6 7 8 9 10	1 2 3 4 5 6 7 8 9 10
Not -------------------------- Extreme	Foggy -------------------------- Clear

How are my bowels?	How is my appetite affected?
1 2 3 4 5 6 7 8 9 10	1 2 3 4 5 6 7 8 9 10
Constipated------------------------- Loose	Not-------------------------- Very

How is my stress level?	How happy am I ?
1 2 3 4 5 6 7 8 9 10	1 2 3 4 5 6 7 8 9 10
None------------------------ Extreme	Not------------------------- Very

Overall pain level?	....
1 2 3 4 5 6 7 8 9 10	1 2 3 4 5 6 7 8 9 10
Low-------------------------- High	--------------------------

TRIGGERS

☐ posture	☐ insomnia	☐ humidity	☐
☐ sleeping	☐ stress	☐ air pressure	☐
☐ exercise	☐ cold/warmth	☐ travel	☐
☐ walking	☐ food	☐ light/sound	☐
☐ weather	☐ lifting	☐ anxiety	☐
☐ allergies	☐ stretching	☐ pms	☐

RELIEF MEASURES

medication	
sleep/rest	
exercise	
Other	

S=Stabbing pain
*= Shooting pain
A=Aching pain
C=Cramping
T=Throbbing Pain
D=Dull pain
N=Numbness
P=Pins and Needles

Mark al the places
that hurt and add
description below

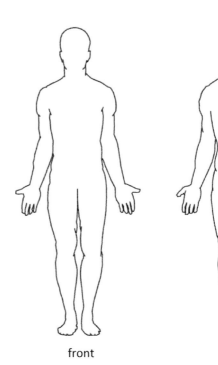

front   back

TIME/ DURATION

	Begin	End	Duration	Description
1				
2				
3				
4				
5				
6				
7				

NOTES (e.g. daily activities, diet, exercise etc.)

DATE	

SYMPTOMS

How well did I sleep?	How energetic do I feel?
1 2 3 4 5 6 7 8 9 10	1 2 3 4 5 6 7 8 9 10
No rest--------------------------- rested	Not --------------------------- Very

How anxious do I feel?	How is my thinking ability
1 2 3 4 5 6 7 8 9 10	1 2 3 4 5 6 7 8 9 10
Not -------------------------- Extreme	Foggy -------------------------- Clear

How are my bowels?	How is my appetite affected?
1 2 3 4 5 6 7 8 9 10	1 2 3 4 5 6 7 8 9 10
Constipated------------------------- Loose	Not--------------------------- Very

How is my stress level?	How happy am I ?
1 2 3 4 5 6 7 8 9 10	1 2 3 4 5 6 7 8 9 10
None------------------------- Extreme	Not-------------------------- Very

Overall pain level?	....
1 2 3 4 5 6 7 8 9 10	1 2 3 4 5 6 7 8 9 10
Low-------------------------- High	---------------------------

TRIGGERS

☐ posture	☐ insomnia	☐ humidity	☐
☐ sleeping	☐ stress	☐ air pressure	☐
☐ exercise	☐ cold/warmth	☐ travel	☐
☐ walking	☐ food	☐ light/sound	☐
☐ weather	☐ lifting	☐ anxiety	☐
☐ allergies	☐ stretching	☐ pms	☐

RELIEF MEASURES

medication	
sleep/rest	
exercise	
Other	

LOCATION

S=Stabbing pain
*= Shooting pain
A=Aching pain
C=Cramping
T=Throbbing Pain
D=Dull pain
N=Numbness
P=Pins and Needles

Mark al the places
that hurt and add
description below

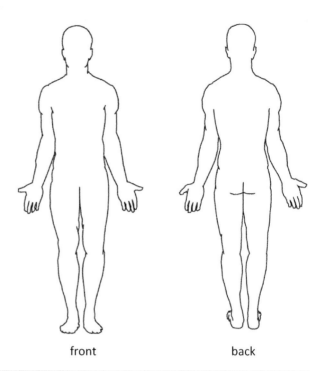

front   back

TIME/ DURATION

	Begin	End	Duration	Description
1				
2				
3				
4				
5				
6				
7				

NOTES (e.g. daily activities, diet, exercise etc.)

SYMPTOMS

How well did I sleep?	How energetic do I feel?
1 2 3 4 5 6 7 8 9 10	1 2 3 4 5 6 7 8 9 10
No rest---------------------------- rested	Not ---------------------------- Very

How anxious do I feel?	How is my thinking ability
1 2 3 4 5 6 7 8 9 10	1 2 3 4 5 6 7 8 9 10
Not -------------------------- Extreme	Foggy -------------------------- Clear

How are my bowels?	How is my appetite affected?
1 2 3 4 5 6 7 8 9 10	1 2 3 4 5 6 7 8 9 10
Constipated------------------------ Loose	Not---------------------------- Very

How is my stress level?	How happy am I ?
1 2 3 4 5 6 7 8 9 10	1 2 3 4 5 6 7 8 9 10
None------------------------ Extreme	Not---------------------------- Very

Overall pain level?	....
1 2 3 4 5 6 7 8 9 10	1 2 3 4 5 6 7 8 9 10
Low-------------------------- High	----------------------------

TRIGGERS

☐ posture	☐ insomnia	☐ humidity	☐
☐ sleeping	☐ stress	☐ air pressure	☐
☐ exercise	☐ cold/warmth	☐ travel	☐
☐ walking	☐ food	☐ light/sound	☐
☐ weather	☐ lifting	☐ anxiety	☐
☐ allergies	☐ stretching	☐ pms	☐

RELIEF MEASURES

medication	
sleep/rest	
exercise	
Other	

LOCATION

S=Stabbing pain
*= Shooting pain
A=Aching pain
C=Cramping
T=Throbbing Pain
D=Dull pain
N=Numbness
P=Pins and Needles

Mark al the places
that hurt and add
description below

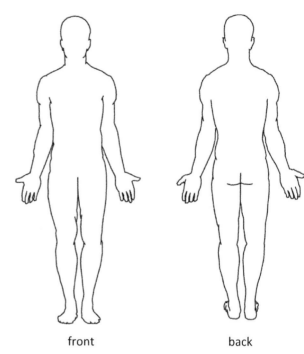

front   back

TIME/ DURATION

	Begin	End	Duration	Description
1				
2				
3				
4				
5				
6				
7				

NOTES (e.g. daily activities, diet, exercise etc.)

SYMPTOMS

How well did I sleep?
1 2 3 4 5 6 7 8 9 10
No rest------------------------- rested

How energetic do I feel?
1 2 3 4 5 6 7 8 9 10
Not ------------------------- Very

How anxious do I feel?
1 2 3 4 5 6 7 8 9 10
Not ------------------------ Extreme

How is my thinking ability
1 2 3 4 5 6 7 8 9 10
Foggy ------------------------- Clear

How are my bowels?
1 2 3 4 5 6 7 8 9 10
Constipated------------------------- Loose

How is my appetite affected?
1 2 3 4 5 6 7 8 9 10
Not------------------------- Very

How is my stress level?
1 2 3 4 5 6 7 8 9 10
None------------------------- Extreme

How happy am I ?
1 2 3 4 5 6 7 8 9 10
Not------------------------ Very

Overall pain level?
1 2 3 4 5 6 7 8 9 10
Low------------------------- High

....
1 2 3 4 5 6 7 8 9 10

TRIGGERS

☐ posture	☐ insomnia	☐ humidity	☐
☐ sleeping	☐ stress	☐ air pressure	☐
☐ exercise	☐ cold/warmth	☐ travel	☐
☐ walking	☐ food	☐ light/sound	☐
☐ weather	☐ lifting	☐ anxiety	☐
☐ allergies	☐ stretching	☐ pms	☐

RELIEF MEASURES

medication	
sleep/rest	
exercise	
Other	

S=Stabbing pain
*= Shooting pain
A=Aching pain
C=Cramping
T=Throbbing Pain
D=Dull pain
N=Numbness
P=Pins and Needles

Mark al the places
that hurt and add
description below

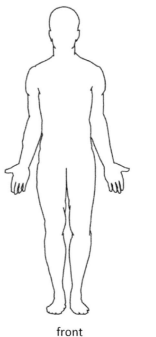
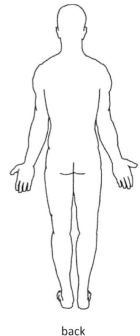

front   back

TIME/ DURATION

	Begin	End	Duration	Description
1				
2				
3				
4				
5				
6				
7				

NOTES (e.g. daily activities, diet, exercise etc.)

DATE	

SYMPTOMS

How well did I sleep?
1 2 3 4 5 6 7 8 9 10
No rest--------------------------- rested

How energetic do I feel?
1 2 3 4 5 6 7 8 9 10
Not --------------------------- Very

How anxious do I feel?
1 2 3 4 5 6 7 8 9 10
Not ------------------------- Extreme

How is my thinking ability
1 2 3 4 5 6 7 8 9 10
Foggy -------------------------- Clear

How are my bowels?
1 2 3 4 5 6 7 8 9 10
Constipated------------------------- Loose

How is my appetite affected?
1 2 3 4 5 6 7 8 9 10
Not--------------------------- Very

How is my stress level?
1 2 3 4 5 6 7 8 9 10
None------------------------- Extreme

How happy am I ?
1 2 3 4 5 6 7 8 9 10
Not--------------------------- Very

Overall pain level?
1 2 3 4 5 6 7 8 9 10
Low-------------------------- High

....
1 2 3 4 5 6 7 8 9 10

TRIGGERS

☐ posture	☐ insomnia	☐ humidity	☐
☐ sleeping	☐ stress	☐ air pressure	☐
☐ exercise	☐ cold/warmth	☐ travel	☐
☐ walking	☐ food	☐ light/sound	☐
☐ weather	☐ lifting	☐ anxiety	☐
☐ allergies	☐ stretching	☐ pms	☐

RELIEF MEASURES

medication	
sleep/rest	
exercise	
Other	

LOCATION

S=Stabbing pain
*= Shooting pain
A=Aching pain
C=Cramping
T=Throbbing Pain
D=Dull pain
N=Numbness
P=Pins and Needles

Mark al the places
that hurt and add
description below

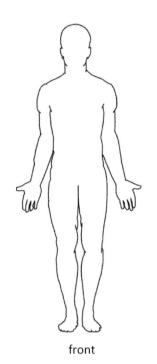
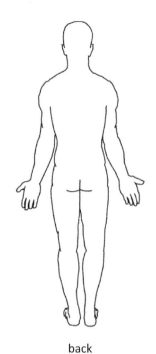

front   back

TIME/ DURATION

	Begin	End	Duration	Description
1				
2				
3				
4				
5				
6				
7				

NOTES (e.g. daily activities, diet, exercise etc.)

SYMPTOMS

How well did I sleep?	How energetic do I feel?
1 2 3 4 5 6 7 8 9 10	1 2 3 4 5 6 7 8 9 10
No rest---------------------------- rested	Not --------------------------- Very

How anxious do I feel?	How is my thinking ability
1 2 3 4 5 6 7 8 9 10	1 2 3 4 5 6 7 8 9 10
Not -------------------------- Extreme	Foggy -------------------------- Clear

How are my bowels?	How is my appetite affected?
1 2 3 4 5 6 7 8 9 10	1 2 3 4 5 6 7 8 9 10
Constipated------------------------ Loose	Not-------------------------- Very

How is my stress level?	How happy am I ?
1 2 3 4 5 6 7 8 9 10	1 2 3 4 5 6 7 8 9 10
None------------------------ Extreme	Not-------------------------- Very

Overall pain level?	....
1 2 3 4 5 6 7 8 9 10	1 2 3 4 5 6 7 8 9 10
Low------------------------- High	----------------------------

TRIGGERS

☐ posture	☐ insomnia	☐ humidity	☐
☐ sleeping	☐ stress	☐ air pressure	☐
☐ exercise	☐ cold/warmth	☐ travel	☐
☐ walking	☐ food	☐ light/sound	☐
☐ weather	☐ lifting	☐ anxiety	☐
☐ allergies	☐ stretching	☐ pms	☐

RELIEF MEASURES

medication	
sleep/rest	
exercise	
Other	

S=Stabbing pain
*= Shooting pain
A=Aching pain
C=Cramping
T=Throbbing Pain
D=Dull pain
N=Numbness
P=Pins and Needles

Mark al the places
that hurt and add
description below

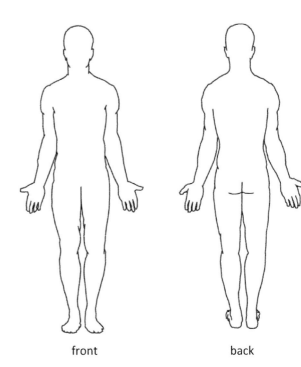

front   back

	Begin	End	Duration	Description
TIME/ DURATION				
1				
2				
3				
4				
5				
6				
7				

NOTES (e.g. daily activities, diet, exercise etc.)

DATE	

SYMPTOMS

How well did I sleep?
1 2 3 4 5 6 7 8 9 10
No rest-------------------------- rested

How energetic do I feel?
1 2 3 4 5 6 7 8 9 10
Not -------------------------- Very

How anxious do I feel?
1 2 3 4 5 6 7 8 9 10
Not -------------------------- Extreme

How is my thinking ability
1 2 3 4 5 6 7 8 9 10
Foggy -------------------------- Clear

How are my bowels?
1 2 3 4 5 6 7 8 9 10
Constipated-------------------------- Loose

How is my appetite affected?
1 2 3 4 5 6 7 8 9 10
Not-------------------------- Very

How is my stress level?
1 2 3 4 5 6 7 8 9 10
None-------------------------- Extreme

How happy am I ?
1 2 3 4 5 6 7 8 9 10
Not-------------------------- Very

Overall pain level?
1 2 3 4 5 6 7 8 9 10
Low-------------------------- High

....
1 2 3 4 5 6 7 8 9 10

TRIGGERS

☐ posture	☐ insomnia	☐ humidity	☐
☐ sleeping	☐ stress	☐ air pressure	☐
☐ exercise	☐ cold/warmth	☐ travel	☐
☐ walking	☐ food	☐ light/sound	☐
☐ weather	☐ lifting	☐ anxiety	☐
☐ allergies	☐ stretching	☐ pms	☐

RELIEF MEASURES

medication	
sleep/rest	
exercise	
Other	

LOCATION

S=Stabbing pain
*= Shooting pain
A=Aching pain
C=Cramping
T=Throbbing Pain
D=Dull pain
N=Numbness
P=Pins and Needles

Mark al the places
that hurt and add
description below

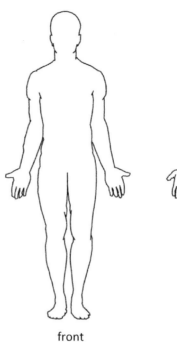 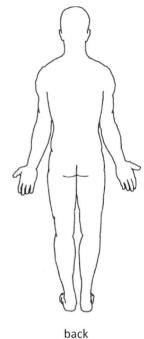

front   back

TIME/ DURATION

	Begin	End	Duration	Description
1				
2				
3				
4				
5				
6				
7				

NOTES (e.g. daily activities, diet, exercise etc.)

DATE	

SYMPTOMS

How well did I sleep?
1 2 3 4 5 6 7 8 9 10
No rest--------------------------- rested

How energetic do I feel?
1 2 3 4 5 6 7 8 9 10
Not --------------------------- Very

How anxious do I feel?
1 2 3 4 5 6 7 8 9 10
Not --------------------------- Extreme

How is my thinking ability
1 2 3 4 5 6 7 8 9 10
Foggy --------------------------- Clear

How are my bowels?
1 2 3 4 5 6 7 8 9 10
Constipated------------------------- Loose

How is my appetite affected?
1 2 3 4 5 6 7 8 9 10
Not--------------------------- Very

How is my stress level?
1 2 3 4 5 6 7 8 9 10
None------------------------- Extreme

How happy am I ?
1 2 3 4 5 6 7 8 9 10
Not--------------------------- Very

Overall pain level?
1 2 3 4 5 6 7 8 9 10
Low------------------------- High

....
1 2 3 4 5 6 7 8 9 10

TRIGGERS

☐ posture	☐ insomnia	☐ humidity	☐
☐ sleeping	☐ stress	☐ air pressure	☐
☐ exercise	☐ cold/warmth	☐ travel	☐
☐ walking	☐ food	☐ light/sound	☐
☐ weather	☐ lifting	☐ anxiety	☐
☐ allergies	☐ stretching	☐ pms	☐

RELIEF MEASURES

medication

sleep/rest

exercise

Other

LOCATION

S=Stabbing pain
*= Shooting pain
A=Aching pain
C=Cramping
T=Throbbing Pain
D=Dull pain
N=Numbness
P=Pins and Needles

Mark al the places
that hurt and add
description below

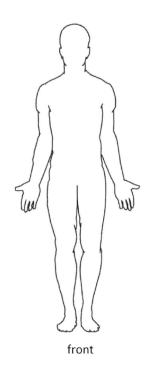
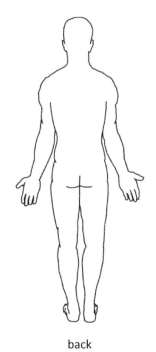

front   back

TIME/ DURATION

	Begin	End	Duration	Description
1				
2				
3				
4				
5				
6				
7				

NOTES (e.g. daily activities, diet, exercise etc.)

SYMPTOMS

How well did I sleep?
1 2 3 4 5 6 7 8 9 10
No rest--------------------------- rested

How energetic do I feel?
1 2 3 4 5 6 7 8 9 10
Not --------------------------- Very

How anxious do I feel?
1 2 3 4 5 6 7 8 9 10
Not --------------------------- Extreme

How is my thinking ability
1 2 3 4 5 6 7 8 9 10
Foggy --------------------------- Clear

How are my bowels?
1 2 3 4 5 6 7 8 9 10
Constipated------------------------- Loose

How is my appetite affected?
1 2 3 4 5 6 7 8 9 10
Not--------------------------- Very

How is my stress level?
1 2 3 4 5 6 7 8 9 10
None------------------------- Extreme

How happy am I ?
1 2 3 4 5 6 7 8 9 10
Not--------------------------- Very

Overall pain level?
1 2 3 4 5 6 7 8 9 10
Low------------------------- High

....
1 2 3 4 5 6 7 8 9 10

TRIGGERS

☐ posture	☐ insomnia	☐ humidity	☐
☐ sleeping	☐ stress	☐ air pressure	☐
☐ exercise	☐ cold/warmth	☐ travel	☐
☐ walking	☐ food	☐ light/sound	☐
☐ weather	☐ lifting	☐ anxiety	☐
☐ allergies	☐ stretching	☐ pms	☐

RELIEF MEASURES

medication

sleep/rest

exercise

Other

S=Stabbing pain
*= Shooting pain
A=Aching pain
C=Cramping
T=Throbbing Pain
D=Dull pain
N=Numbness
P=Pins and Needles

Mark al the places
that hurt and add
description below

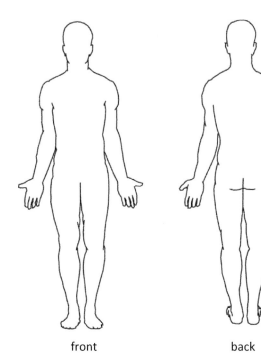

front   back

TIME/ DURATION

	Begin	End	Duration	Description
1				
2				
3				
4				
5				
6				
7				

NOTES (e.g. daily activities, diet, exercise etc.)

DATE	

SYMPTOMS

How well did I sleep?	How energetic do I feel?
1 2 3 4 5 6 7 8 9 10	1 2 3 4 5 6 7 8 9 10
No rest-------------------------- rested	Not --------------------------- Very

How anxious do I feel?	How is my thinking ability
1 2 3 4 5 6 7 8 9 10	1 2 3 4 5 6 7 8 9 10
Not -------------------------- Extreme	Foggy ------------------------- Clear

How are my bowels?	How is my appetite affected?
1 2 3 4 5 6 7 8 9 10	1 2 3 4 5 6 7 8 9 10
Constipated------------------------- Loose	Not--------------------------- Very

How is my stress level?	How happy am I ?
1 2 3 4 5 6 7 8 9 10	1 2 3 4 5 6 7 8 9 10
None------------------------- Extreme	Not--------------------------- Very

Overall pain level?	....
1 2 3 4 5 6 7 8 9 10	1 2 3 4 5 6 7 8 9 10
Low-------------------------- High	---------------------------

TRIGGERS

☐ posture	☐ insomnia	☐ humidity	☐
☐ sleeping	☐ stress	☐ air pressure	☐
☐ exercise	☐ cold/warmth	☐ travel	☐
☐ walking	☐ food	☐ light/sound	☐
☐ weather	☐ lifting	☐ anxiety	☐
☐ allergies	☐ stretching	☐ pms	☐

RELIEF MEASURES

medication	
sleep/rest	
exercise	
Other	

LOCATION

S=Stabbing pain
*= Shooting pain
A=Aching pain
C=Cramping
T=Throbbing Pain
D=Dull pain
N=Numbness
P=Pins and Needles

Mark al the places
that hurt and add
description below

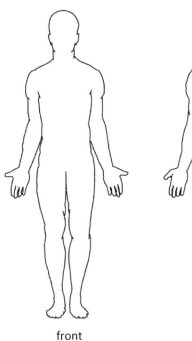
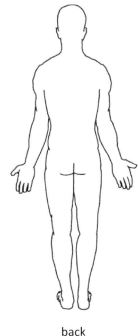

front   back

TIME/ DURATION

	Begin	End	Duration	Description
1				
2				
3				
4				
5				
6				
7				

NOTES (e.g. daily activities, diet, exercise etc.)

DATE	

SYMPTOMS

How well did I sleep?
1 2 3 4 5 6 7 8 9 10
No rest-------------------------- rested

How energetic do I feel?
1 2 3 4 5 6 7 8 9 10
Not --------------------------- Very

How anxious do I feel?
1 2 3 4 5 6 7 8 9 10
Not --------------------------- Extreme

How is my thinking ability
1 2 3 4 5 6 7 8 9 10
Foggy --------------------------- Clear

How are my bowels?
1 2 3 4 5 6 7 8 9 10
Constipated------------------------- Loose

How is my appetite affected?
1 2 3 4 5 6 7 8 9 10
Not--------------------------- Very

How is my stress level?
1 2 3 4 5 6 7 8 9 10
None----------------------- Extreme

How happy am I ?
1 2 3 4 5 6 7 8 9 10
Not------------------------- Very

Overall pain level?
1 2 3 4 5 6 7 8 9 10
Low------------------------- High

....
1 2 3 4 5 6 7 8 9 10

TRIGGERS

☐ posture	☐ insomnia	☐ humidity	☐
☐ sleeping	☐ stress	☐ air pressure	☐
☐ exercise	☐ cold/warmth	☐ travel	☐
☐ walking	☐ food	☐ light/sound	☐
☐ weather	☐ lifting	☐ anxiety	☐
☐ allergies	☐ stretching	☐ pms	☐

RELIEF MEASURES

medication	
sleep/rest	
exercise	
Other	

S=Stabbing pain
*= Shooting pain
A=Aching pain
C=Cramping
T=Throbbing Pain
D=Dull pain
N=Numbness
P=Pins and Needles

Mark al the places
that hurt and add
description below

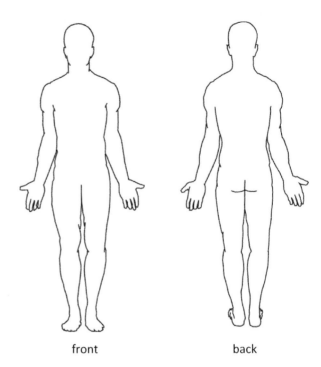

front   back

TIME/ DURATION

	Begin	End	Duration	Description
1				
2				
3				
4				
5				
6				
7				

NOTES (e.g. daily activities, diet, exercise etc.)

SYMPTOMS

How well did I sleep?
1 2 3 4 5 6 7 8 9 10
No rest---------------------------- rested

How energetic do I feel?
1 2 3 4 5 6 7 8 9 10
Not ---------------------------- Very

How anxious do I feel?
1 2 3 4 5 6 7 8 9 10
Not ------------------------- Extreme

How is my thinking ability
1 2 3 4 5 6 7 8 9 10
Foggy ------------------------- Clear

How are my bowels?
1 2 3 4 5 6 7 8 9 10
Constipated------------------------- Loose

How is my appetite affected?
1 2 3 4 5 6 7 8 9 10
Not------------------------- Very

How is my stress level?
1 2 3 4 5 6 7 8 9 10
None------------------------- Extreme

How happy am I ?
1 2 3 4 5 6 7 8 9 10
Not------------------------- Very

Overall pain level?
1 2 3 4 5 6 7 8 9 10
Low------------------------- High

....
1 2 3 4 5 6 7 8 9 10

TRIGGERS

☐ posture   ☐ insomnia   ☐ humidity   ☐
☐ sleeping   ☐ stress   ☐ air pressure ☐
☐ exercise   ☐ cold/warmth ☐ travel   ☐
☐ walking   ☐ food   ☐ light/sound ☐
☐ weather   ☐ lifting   ☐ anxiety   ☐
☐ allergies ☐ stretching ☐ pms   ☐

RELIEF MEASURES

medication

sleep/rest

exercise

Other

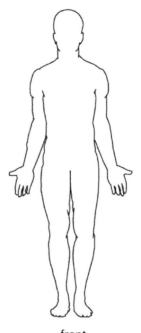 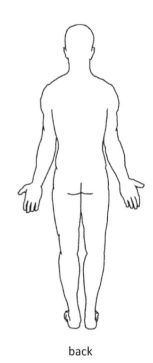

front   back

	Begin	End	Duration	Description
TIME/ DURATION				
1				
2				
3				
4				
5				
6				
7				

NOTES (e.g. daily activities, diet, exercise etc.)

SYMPTOMS

How well did I sleep?	How energetic do I feel?
1 2 3 4 5 6 7 8 9 10	1 2 3 4 5 6 7 8 9 10
No rest---------------------------- rested	Not ---------------------------- Very

How anxious do I feel?	How is my thinking ability
1 2 3 4 5 6 7 8 9 10	1 2 3 4 5 6 7 8 9 10
Not --------------------------- Extreme	Foggy ---------------------------- Clear

How are my bowels?	How is my appetite affected?
1 2 3 4 5 6 7 8 9 10	1 2 3 4 5 6 7 8 9 10
Constipated------------------------- Loose	Not---------------------------- Very

How is my stress level?	How happy am I ?
1 2 3 4 5 6 7 8 9 10	1 2 3 4 5 6 7 8 9 10
None------------------------ Extreme	Not---------------------------- Very

Overall pain level?	....
1 2 3 4 5 6 7 8 9 10	1 2 3 4 5 6 7 8 9 10
Low------------------------- High	----------------------------

TRIGGERS

☐ posture	☐ insomnia	☐ humidity	☐
☐ sleeping	☐ stress	☐ air pressure	☐
☐ exercise	☐ cold/warmth	☐ travel	☐
☐ walking	☐ food	☐ light/sound	☐
☐ weather	☐ lifting	☐ anxiety	☐
☐ allergies	☐ stretching	☐ pms	☐

RELIEF MEASURES

medication	
sleep/rest	
exercise	
Other	

LOCATION

S=Stabbing pain
*= Shooting pain
A=Aching pain
C=Cramping
T=Throbbing Pain
D=Dull pain
N=Numbness
P=Pins and Needles

Mark al the places
that hurt and add
description below

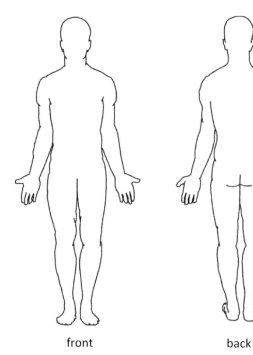

front   back

TIME/ DURATION

	Begin	End	Duration	Description
1				
2				
3				
4				
5				
6				
7				

NOTES (e.g. daily activities, diet, exercise etc.)

DATE	

SYMPTOMS

How well did I sleep?

1 2 3 4 5 6 7 8 9 10
No rest-------------------------- rested

How energetic do I feel?

1 2 3 4 5 6 7 8 9 10
Not -------------------------- Very

How anxious do I feel?

1 2 3 4 5 6 7 8 9 10
Not -------------------------- Extreme

How is my thinking ability

1 2 3 4 5 6 7 8 9 10
Foggy -------------------------- Clear

How are my bowels?

1 2 3 4 5 6 7 8 9 10
Constipated------------------------- Loose

How is my appetite affected?

1 2 3 4 5 6 7 8 9 10
Not-------------------------- Very

How is my stress level?

1 2 3 4 5 6 7 8 9 10
None------------------------- Extreme

How happy am I ?

1 2 3 4 5 6 7 8 9 10
Not-------------------------- Very

Overall pain level?

1 2 3 4 5 6 7 8 9 10
Low------------------------- High

....
1 2 3 4 5 6 7 8 9 10

TRIGGERS

☐ posture	☐ insomnia	☐ humidity	☐
☐ sleeping	☐ stress	☐ air pressure	☐
☐ exercise	☐ cold/warmth	☐ travel	☐
☐ walking	☐ food	☐ light/sound	☐
☐ weather	☐ lifting	☐ anxiety	☐
☐ allergies	☐ stretching	☐ pms	☐

RELIEF MEASURES

medication

sleep/rest

exercise

Other

S=Stabbing pain
*= Shooting pain
A=Aching pain
C=Cramping
T=Throbbing Pain
D=Dull pain
N=Numbness
P=Pins and Needles

Mark al the places
that hurt and add
description below

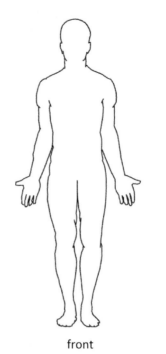 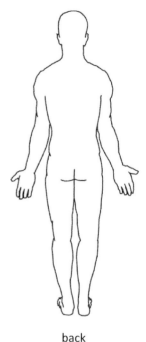

front   back

TIME/ DURATION

	Begin	End	Duration	Description
1				
2				
3				
4				
5				
6				
7				

NOTES (e.g. daily activities, diet, exercise etc.)

DATE	

SYMPTOMS

How well did I sleep?
1 2 3 4 5 6 7 8 9 10
No rest-------------------------- rested

How energetic do I feel?
1 2 3 4 5 6 7 8 9 10
Not -------------------------- Very

How anxious do I feel?
1 2 3 4 5 6 7 8 9 10
Not -------------------------- Extreme

How is my thinking ability
1 2 3 4 5 6 7 8 9 10
Foggy -------------------------- Clear

How are my bowels?
1 2 3 4 5 6 7 8 9 10
Constipated------------------------ Loose

How is my appetite affected?
1 2 3 4 5 6 7 8 9 10
Not-------------------------- Very

How is my stress level?
1 2 3 4 5 6 7 8 9 10
None------------------------ Extreme

How happy am I ?
1 2 3 4 5 6 7 8 9 10
Not-------------------------- Very

Overall pain level?
1 2 3 4 5 6 7 8 9 10
Low-------------------------- High

....
1 2 3 4 5 6 7 8 9 10

TRIGGERS

☐ posture	☐ insomnia	☐ humidity	☐
☐ sleeping	☐ stress	☐ air pressure	☐
☐ exercise	☐ cold/warmth	☐ travel	☐
☐ walking	☐ food	☐ light/sound	☐
☐ weather	☐ lifting	☐ anxiety	☐
☐ allergies	☐ stretching	☐ pms	☐

RELIEF MEASURES

medication	
sleep/rest	
exercise	
Other	

S=Stabbing pain
*= Shooting pain
A=Aching pain
C=Cramping
T=Throbbing Pain
D=Dull pain
N=Numbness
P=Pins and Needles

Mark al the places
that hurt and add
description below

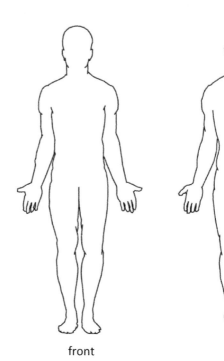

front   back

TIME/ DURATION

	Begin	End	Duration	Description
1				
2				
3				
4				
5				
6				
7				

NOTES (e.g. daily activities, diet, exercise etc.)

SYMPTOMS

How well did I sleep?
1 2 3 4 5 6 7 8 9 10
No rest-------------------------- rested

How energetic do I feel?
1 2 3 4 5 6 7 8 9 10
Not -------------------------- Very

How anxious do I feel?
1 2 3 4 5 6 7 8 9 10
Not -------------------------- Extreme

How is my thinking ability
1 2 3 4 5 6 7 8 9 10
Foggy -------------------------- Clear

How are my bowels?
1 2 3 4 5 6 7 8 9 10
Constipated------------------------- Loose

How is my appetite affected?
1 2 3 4 5 6 7 8 9 10
Not-------------------------- Very

How is my stress level?
1 2 3 4 5 6 7 8 9 10
None------------------------- Extreme

How happy am I ?
1 2 3 4 5 6 7 8 9 10
Not-------------------------- Very

Overall pain level?
1 2 3 4 5 6 7 8 9 10
Low-------------------------- High

....
1 2 3 4 5 6 7 8 9 10

TRIGGERS

☐ posture	☐ insomnia	☐ humidity	☐
☐ sleeping	☐ stress	☐ air pressure	☐
☐ exercise	☐ cold/warmth	☐ travel	☐
☐ walking	☐ food	☐ light/sound	☐
☐ weather	☐ lifting	☐ anxiety	☐
☐ allergies	☐ stretching	☐ pms	☐

RELIEF MEASURES

medication	
sleep/rest	
exercise	
Other	

LOCATION

S=Stabbing pain
*= Shooting pain
A=Aching pain
C=Cramping
T=Throbbing Pain
D=Dull pain
N=Numbness
P=Pins and Needles

Mark al the places
that hurt and add
description below

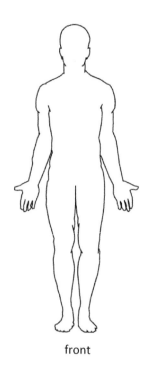
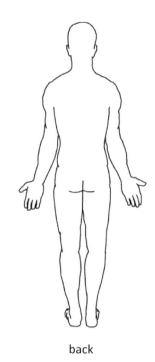

front   back

TIME/ DURATION

	Begin	End	Duration	Description
1				
2				
3				
4				
5				
6				
7				

NOTES (e.g. daily activities, diet, exercise etc.)

DATE	

SYMPTOMS

How well did I sleep?
1 2 3 4 5 6 7 8 9 10
No rest--------------------------- rested

How energetic do I feel?
1 2 3 4 5 6 7 8 9 10
Not --------------------------- Very

How anxious do I feel?
1 2 3 4 5 6 7 8 9 10
Not --------------------------- Extreme

How is my thinking ability
1 2 3 4 5 6 7 8 9 10
Foggy --------------------------- Clear

How are my bowels?
1 2 3 4 5 6 7 8 9 10
Constipated------------------------- Loose

How is my appetite affected?
1 2 3 4 5 6 7 8 9 10
Not--------------------------- Very

How is my stress level?
1 2 3 4 5 6 7 8 9 10
None------------------------- Extreme

How happy am I ?
1 2 3 4 5 6 7 8 9 10
Not--------------------------- Very

Overall pain level?
1 2 3 4 5 6 7 8 9 10
Low------------------------- High

....
1 2 3 4 5 6 7 8 9 10

TRIGGERS

☐ posture	☐ insomnia	☐ humidity	☐
☐ sleeping	☐ stress	☐ air pressure	☐
☐ exercise	☐ cold/warmth	☐ travel	☐
☐ walking	☐ food	☐ light/sound	☐
☐ weather	☐ lifting	☐ anxiety	☐
☐ allergies	☐ stretching	☐ pms	☐

RELIEF MEASURES

medication	
sleep/rest	
exercise	
Other	

LOCATION

S=Stabbing pain
*= Shooting pain
A=Aching pain
C=Cramping
T=Throbbing Pain
D=Dull pain
N=Numbness
P=Pins and Needles

Mark al the places
that hurt and add
description below

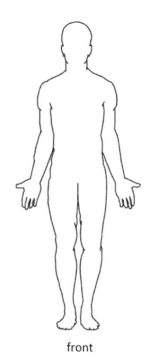

front

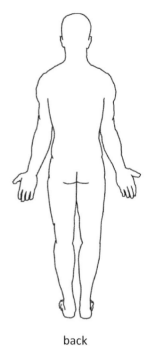

back

TIME/ DURATION

	Begin	End	Duration	Description
1				
2				
3				
4				
5				
6				
7				

NOTES (e.g. daily activities, diet, exercise etc.)

SYMPTOMS

How well did I sleep?
1 2 3 4 5 6 7 8 9 10
No rest---------------------------- rested

How energetic do I feel?
1 2 3 4 5 6 7 8 9 10
Not --------------------------- Very

How anxious do I feel?
1 2 3 4 5 6 7 8 9 10
Not ------------------------- Extreme

How is my thinking ability
1 2 3 4 5 6 7 8 9 10
Foggy -------------------------- Clear

How are my bowels?
1 2 3 4 5 6 7 8 9 10
Constipated------------------------ Loose

How is my appetite affected?
1 2 3 4 5 6 7 8 9 10
Not--------------------------- Very

How is my stress level?
1 2 3 4 5 6 7 8 9 10
None------------------------ Extreme

How happy am I ?
1 2 3 4 5 6 7 8 9 10
Not--------------------------- Very

Overall pain level?
1 2 3 4 5 6 7 8 9 10
Low------------------------- High

....
1 2 3 4 5 6 7 8 9 10

TRIGGERS

☐ posture	☐ insomnia	☐ humidity	☐
☐ sleeping	☐ stress	☐ air pressure	☐
☐ exercise	☐ cold/warmth	☐ travel	☐
☐ walking	☐ food	☐ light/sound	☐
☐ weather	☐ lifting	☐ anxiety	☐
☐ allergies	☐ stretching	☐ pms	☐

RELIEF MEASURES

medication

sleep/rest

exercise

Other

S=Stabbing pain
*= Shooting pain
A=Aching pain
C=Cramping
T=Throbbing Pain
D=Dull pain
N=Numbness
P=Pins and Needles

Mark al the places
that hurt and add
description below

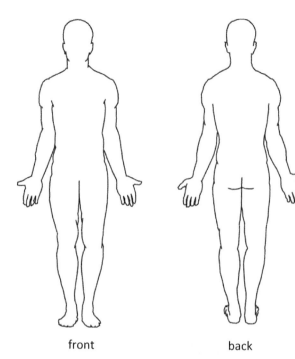

front   back

TIME/ DURATION

	Begin	End	Duration	Description
1				
2				
3				
4				
5				
6				
7				

NOTES (e.g. daily activities, diet, exercise etc.)

SYMPTOMS

How well did I sleep?	How energetic do I feel?
1 2 3 4 5 6 7 8 9 10	1 2 3 4 5 6 7 8 9 10
No rest---------------------------- rested	Not ---------------------------- Very

How anxious do I feel?	How is my thinking ability
1 2 3 4 5 6 7 8 9 10	1 2 3 4 5 6 7 8 9 10
Not ---------------------------- Extreme	Foggy ---------------------------- Clear

How are my bowels?	How is my appetite affected?
1 2 3 4 5 6 7 8 9 10	1 2 3 4 5 6 7 8 9 10
Constipated------------------------- Loose	Not---------------------------- Very

How is my stress level?	How happy am I ?
1 2 3 4 5 6 7 8 9 10	1 2 3 4 5 6 7 8 9 10
None------------------------- Extreme	Not---------------------------- Very

Overall pain level?	....
1 2 3 4 5 6 7 8 9 10	1 2 3 4 5 6 7 8 9 10
Low------------------------- High	----------------------------

TRIGGERS

☐ posture	☐ insomnia	☐ humidity	☐
☐ sleeping	☐ stress	☐ air pressure	☐
☐ exercise	☐ cold/warmth	☐ travel	☐
☐ walking	☐ food	☐ light/sound	☐
☐ weather	☐ lifting	☐ anxiety	☐
☐ allergies	☐ stretching	☐ pms	☐

RELIEF MEASURES

medication	
sleep/rest	
exercise	
Other	

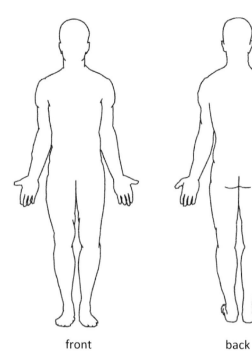

front   back

TIME/ DURATION

	Begin	End	Duration	Description
1				
2				
3				
4				
5				
6				
7				

NOTES (e.g. daily activities, diet, exercise etc.)

	DATE	

SYMPTOMS

How well did I sleep?	How energetic do I feel?
1 2 3 4 5 6 7 8 9 10	1 2 3 4 5 6 7 8 9 10
No rest---------------------------- rested	Not ---------------------------- Very

How anxious do I feel?	How is my thinking ability
1 2 3 4 5 6 7 8 9 10	1 2 3 4 5 6 7 8 9 10
Not -------------------------- Extreme	Foggy -------------------------- Clear

How are my bowels?	How is my appetite affected?
1 2 3 4 5 6 7 8 9 10	1 2 3 4 5 6 7 8 9 10
Constipated------------------------- Loose	Not-------------------------- Very

How is my stress level?	How happy am I ?
1 2 3 4 5 6 7 8 9 10	1 2 3 4 5 6 7 8 9 10
None------------------------- Extreme	Not-------------------------- Very

Overall pain level?	....
1 2 3 4 5 6 7 8 9 10	1 2 3 4 5 6 7 8 9 10
Low------------------------- High	-----------------------------

TRIGGERS

☐ posture	☐ insomnia	☐ humidity	☐
☐ sleeping	☐ stress	☐ air pressure	☐
☐ exercise	☐ cold/warmth	☐ travel	☐
☐ walking	☐ food	☐ light/sound	☐
☐ weather	☐ lifting	☐ anxiety	☐
☐ allergies	☐ stretching	☐ pms	☐

RELIEF MEASURES

medication	
sleep/rest	
exercise	
Other	

Printed in Great Britain
by Amazon